LOST IN COGNITION

LOST IN COGNITION
Psychoanalysis and the Cognitive Sciences

Éric Laurent

Translated from the French by A. R. Price

KARNAC

Originally published in French by Éditions Cécile Defaut © MMVIII

First published in English in 2014 by
Karnac Books Ltd
118 Finchley Road
London NW3 5HT

British Library Cataloguing in Publication Data

A C.I.P. for this book is available from the British Library

ISBN-13: 978-1-78220-088-8

Typeset by V Publishing Solutions Pvt Ltd., Chennai, India

Printed in Great Britain

www.karnacbooks.com

CONTENTS

ABOUT THE AUTHOR

Éric Laurent is a former president of the World Association of Psychoanalysis and author of *La bataille de l'autisme: de la clinique à la politique*. In 2004, he delivered the "Eight Guiding Principles for Any Psychoanalytic Act" to the General Assembly of the WAP, and, in 2011, he was invited to deliver the Abram Kardiner Lecture at the New York Academy of Medicine. Éric Laurent has lectured widely in Europe, Israel, and Latin America, and his articles are regularly translated into English in *Psychoanalytical Notebooks*, *Lacanian Ink* and *Hurly-Burly*.

Loss and cognition

This book examines the pretensions of the new paradigm in psychology, a paradigm that has been pushed to the fore as the model for the future of clinical disciplines in the hope of thereby putting paid to psychoanalysis. What is this paradigm shift? It goes by the name of cognitive behaviourism and comes from the United States. Until the 1960s, behavioural psychology had enjoyed a certain prestige in the US. It was later discredited by objections from the linguist Noam Chomsky who held that no learning procedure could ever account for linguistic competence. This competence was surely innate, argued Chomsky, and so he set about hunting out the organ of language. Behaviour would have to be complemented by *a machine for taking cognisance*, an innate machine that conformed to the post-Chomskyan model. It took the discipline some thirty years to deck itself out in new clothes. The advances in biology, in neurology, and in the resulting nebula under the "neuroscience" label, oversaw this change.

Synonymies abound in academic cognitivist neo-speak. They give rise to ambiguity of sufficient scale to support a community. The 1931 publication of Paul Valéry's *Reflections on the World Today* included the 1927 "Notes on the greatness and decadence of Europe", in which we find a definition of "nation" that, for Valéry, is at once a powerful and indefinable notion.

> Yet when men use these indefinable terms among themselves, they understand each other very well. These notions are, then, clear and adequate between man and man, but obscure and almost infinitely conflicting in each man taken by himself. (Valéry, 1951, p. 33)

Only vague symbols can approach this bond, a bond formed in the drive and located beyond clear and distinct concepts.

This same extension is what allows us to speak with one other, and then, when we need greater precision, science makes an appearance. Science too creates a language, but it does not target the social bond.

The essential feature of this neo-speak is that it has the widest possible array of synonymies at its disposal, and they have allowed a conversation to be established between former-Chomskyans, neurologists, biologists, and academics. It gives the impression that they are speaking with each other about something they have in common when they are actually speaking about things that are rather different. This conversation held in the name of science is a pure social bond, a semblance of science.

Cognitivist neo-speak has spread quickly, coinciding with a generational shift amongst psychiatrists and psychologists. It is now looking to become more firmly entrenched. The common ideology, or rather the common hope, of academic psychology today is to try to reduce the subject of psychology to a system of learning. It is both executing and exceeding Piaget's programme of unifying psychology around a behavioural vision of children's learning, whilst giving up on references to logic and language.

It is not just academic psychology that is being recast by the cognitive-behavioural project. From the start, this project opted for the US classification of mental illnesses programme that came to be generalised in the *Diagnostic and Statistical Manual of Mental Disorders* (DSM). The two programmes do not overlap entirely, but there is considerable crossover. The cognitive-behavioural perspective is presented as the solution to the difficulties that the DSM met in wanting to reduce psychopathology to elementary data that could be fully observed with no leftovers. The recent publication of the fifth edition of the DSM has given rise to debates that indicate an impasse has been reached. The cognitive-behavioural project will emerge from this in altered form. We shall see how in the epilogue that has been added specially for this English-language edition.

The different modalities by which experience is inscribed in the nervous system, by virtue of the latter's "plasticity", have restored the learning model to favour. Under the name of behavioural cognitivism, a new reduction of human experience to learning has emerged.

In its descriptive accounts it leans not only on behaviour observation but also on the cerebral imagery that can be obtained by means of magnetic resonance imaging (MRI) and position emission tomography (PET scanning). By virtue of the commentary it gives on these images the new psychology claims to hold a legitimate place among the neurosciences.

Some psychoanalysts have been encouraging colleagues to follow the same path that psychology has taken, arguing that there will be a place for the Freudian unconscious processes amongst the diversity of models of cognition. Some think that the time has come for subjective processes to be translated in terms of neuronal networks. This is the error of the theoreticians of cognitivism and the supporters of cognitive psychoanalysis, both of whom think that neuroscience in fact merely confirms the discoveries of Freud and Lacan.

Based on the psychoanalysis of Lacanian orientation this book upholds an opposing thesis: what has been lost in this would-be translation is the unconscious itself. We lose sight of the subject of the analytic experience and the object of psychoanalysis.

The unconscious does not fall into the category of "learning". It is what is *missing from* or *surplus to* any possible learning process. After all that has been learnt during the day, the dream awakens on the basis of that which has not been learnt, uttered, or thought. The unconscious is a mode of thought free from both learning and consciousness, and this is what is at once odd and scandalous about it. We maintain that there is a fundamental disjunction between what would amount to a subject determined by his learning processes (regardless of the more or less sophisticated conception one may have of learning) and a subject determined by the unconscious. The unconscious does not allow itself to be cut down to the size of a learning system, or traces of learning. What are presumed to be traces enter a topological system that is formed in such a way that they cannot be inscribed onto a surface (for instance, the surface of the neuronal cortex). Only the topology of the letter can account for this. Lacan's topology stands in opposition to any conception of a system of traces inscribed on a surface that could be mapped. It matters little here whether one thinks of synaptic connections in terms of a network (like the GSM model of the global system for mobile communication) or in terms of a constellation of satellites (constituting a Global Positioning System that would one day allow everyone to be located with perfect precision). Both perspectives are at odds with the viewpoint of an unconscious that is understood as the deposit of the equivocations of all possible languages.

Equivocation is one of the names for the impossibility of deducing a subject from the traces of any given experience. This is an impossible relation because the subject always ends up mistakenly connecting himself to other traces.

A subject determined by equivocations implies a break from learning processes. We are constantly running up against the impossibility of getting back to anything that might amount to an originative trace. In other words, we always meet the *Tuchē*, which is not a trace of learning but a missed encounter, as Lacan explains. There is always equivocation with respect to what actually occurred.

Not only is it impossible to get back to the original trace, but also a finite number of learning processes cannot generate an infinite system of equivocations, sentences, languages, and so forth.

Before the neurosciences, one of Lacan's pupils had tried to put forward a model of the unconscious reduced to a system of "learnings"; erotic "learnings" no doubt, but "learnings" all the same. That pupil was Serge Leclaire. He was of the idea that one could form a conception of the unconscious in terms of traces inscribed onto an erogenous body. Combined with one another, these *erotic traces* would ostensibly link up with language. But Leclaire kept running into the same problem: if the system of any given language is infinite, what are the systems that allow us to pass from a system in which there is a finite battery to a system that is infinite? Something does not sit right here. The locus of the subject is required as a Russellian set that articulates the two systems. There is no compatibility between the subject as a Russellian set and the subject of learning. The property of neuronal plasticity, far from authorising any depositing of all possible traces, seals with the mark of impossibility the programme that seeks to reduce experience to its trace.

What has been lost in the cognitive stance—*lost in cognition*—is the originality of the Freudian unconscious. Precipitated from speech, this unconscious finds its locus in a written form and not in traces. Its locus lies outside the body. It is articulated to the body of living beings, however, by experiences of jouissance that remain unforgettable. The three sections that make up this book seek to demonstrate this articulation.

The first section opens by examining the status of the unconscious as exemplified by Joyce's text and how Lacan relates it to Chomsky's conception of the language module. The term "cognitivism" covers very different programmes. Chomsky's cognitivism is one thing, the cognitive therapies are quite another. The two programmes have nothing to do with each other. Lacan's reflection opens a dialogue with Chomsky's programme and opposes it. To think that what languages have in common is that they allow for the emergence of science is quite different from thinking that what they have in common is generative grammar in the form of a language organ. Lacan's reflection strikes me as decisive. The Lacanian perspective consists rather in postulating clearly that what languages have in common is not grammar but the possibility of science. Natural languages convey number, and number is what then allows for the emergence of science.

The second article looks at the impossibility of reducing the subject to traces of learning processes. In particular, we pursue a dialogue with Pierre Magistretti and François Ansermet who offer an original solution to link neuroscience and psychoanalysis. In a book published in 2004,[1] they take on board the accepted notion of "psychical trace", but accentuate plasticity rather than the trace itself. They call into question the notion of the brain reduced to a pure automaton of traces by considering not only inscription in the cortex but also inscription in the body: the somato-psychical bond. Thus, they reject any fixed correspondence between an emotion and a bodily state. We accept their thesis that there is a space for renewed inscriptions of synapses and that in this sense one never uses the same brain twice. On the other hand, it remains the case that there is a radical impossibility of reducing subjective inscription to a system of traces.

The second section broaches a further point of impossibility, which stems from the first: that of evaluation when it seeks to reduce the particularity of the subjective symptom by apportioning it into tick-boxes. The mad machine of the ideology of evaluation is striving to turn everything into a uniform entity, with all the psychotherapies and every which treatment technique translated into a kind of universal code by means of a procedure that implements an all-pervasive assessment of these practices. The first article examines the failures of a project by France's *Institut national de la santé et de la recherche médicale* (Inserm) when in 2004 it evaluated the psychotherapies using an inappropriate model that homogenised each of the various therapeutic practices. The subsequent 2005 assessments on "conduct disorder in children and adolescents" ended up triggering a strong reaction of rejection in the form of the *pas de zéro de conduite* petition. This evaluative machinery run amok is examined here in its precise functioning. The problem resides in the connection between *state apparatus* and its *sanitary bureaucracy* couched in the language of cognitivist evaluation. The connection between this neo-speak and the rhetoric of evaluation is the infernal machine that today constitutes our environment and the very air we breathe. It constitutes an apparatus that strives to scale down the space in which the subject dwells, namely, the space of *equivocation*. There is an ongoing effort to reduce the subject to his skills, to his social abilities, and to his knowledge-learning competence, that is, to conditions for potential learning.

The third section groups together three assorted papers. The first, "On the origin of the Other and the post-traumatic object", is addressed to those post-Chomskyans who have been attempting to find a modality of the origin of language beyond the dividing line between animal species and humans. For psychoanalysis of Lacanian orientation, the cut that Lévi-Strauss accentuated between nature and culture is displaced. Lacan proposes something different: that psychoanalysis leaves behind the animal-human opposition in favour of that between the living being and the speaking being.

The second article examines the state of cognitivist psychoanalysis, the monster born of this attempt to translate psychoanalytic hypotheses by taking a detour via cognitivism. The mainstream of psychoanalysis in the US today is the former ego psychology current translated into cognitive terms. The ego-psychoanalysts now use the language of neuroscientist and physiologist of memory, Eric Kandel, or of emotional cognitivist Antonio Damasio. They maintain that in order to survive as a scientific discipline, one must use cognitivist jargon; and they apply this policy to both psychology and psychiatry. They assert that not only must one use the language of the DSM to maintain a dialogue with psychiatrists, but also one must adopt the classification by disorders rather than by symptoms. This has led them to renounce psychoanalysis, as we show in our examples.

In opposition to this standpoint we set out what is most specific to the analytic discourse. This discourse situates the specific real of psychoanalysis, in which one encounters the subject of its experience. The symptom turns out to be untranslatable in terms of *disorder*, when the latter is understood as a cognitive error. The dimension of the particularity of the subject of the symptom can be contrasted with the homogenising category of disorder (as a cognitive error). For example, the latter category generalises the conception of hallucination as an error of perception. Lacan was against such an approach and showed that, far from being a perceptual error, a hallucination is a manifestation of the subject's truth. The term "cognition" has fallen prey to a great deal of loose talk, notably some unfortunate synonymies, but there is no cause to go running to the neurosciences, making out that they say the same thing as psychoanalysis or that they confirm it. We ought rather to single out two planes: the plane of scientific objectivity and the plane of the objectality of psychoanalysis. *Scientific objectivity* and *psychoanalytic objectality* are fundamentally heterogeneous. Indeed, the object *a*, the notorious object constructed by Lacan as *Dasein*, the subject's Being, cannot be demonstrated by science. Starting off from the object *a* and the symptom, we must examine both the effect science has on the way the subject is produced and the regime of scientific certainties. The principles of Lacanian analytic practice ground interpretation upon the experience of a real that is specific to psychoanalysis, and not upon any conformity with the objects produced by a scientific discourse.

Lastly, an epilogue examines the consequences of the failure of the DSM programme and the new configurations that are being produced to replace it. The cognitive-behavioural programme is now being modified by the newly affirmed scientific necessity of bypassing the observation of behaviour, and we are seeing new clinical research programmes that seek to observe biomarkers. The study of behaviour has lost its prestige and there is now a general wariness about authoritarian behaviour modification. The article "The new pathways of loss in the DSM-5 impasse" examines how the cards are being re-dealt to the various players in the clinical field whose divergent interests are not about to converge anytime soon in a unifying paradigm. Something new is going to remain "lost in cognition".

Éric Laurent

Note

1. The English-language translation appeared three years later (Ansermet & Magistretti, 2007).

PART I

HOW IS THE SUBJECT INSCRIBED?

CHAPTER ONE

Chomsky with Joyce

The following lecture was delivered at the École de la Cause freudienne on 11 April 2005. Under Serge Cottet's chairmanship, Jacques Aubert and Éric Laurent were invited to present the recently published Book of Lacan's Seminar, Le Sinthome.

When you look at Jacques Lacan's admirable *Seminar XXIII* in the form it has now found,[1] with its superb and serene knots, matched up with Lacan's 1975 lecture, with the surprising "Reading notes" by Jacques Aubert, and finally with Jacques-Alain Miller's "Note threaded stitch by stitch", one can scarcely imagine our dread back then as we sat in the audience of Lacan's Seminar.

In November 1975, we could but take measure of our unfathomable ignorance.

First of all, there was Joyce, whom we thought we had read when we were younger. We knew that this was just a first entry into reading Joyce, but we did think we had crossed the threshold. Now all of a sudden we found ourselves back on the outside. We simply weren't on the right page. We would have to start from scratch. It was "all hands on deck" to try to get hold of a copy of the Viking Press edition of *Finnegans*

Wake, which wasn't easy to come by. The Richard Ellmann biography was essential reading, as were a host of other items.

Our first impression was that this was a vast undertaking. And what about the knots! And the diagrams! How would we ever make head or tail of it? We formed work groups, cartels. The blind leading the paralytic. We soon got through the available books on the knots—there weren't many at the time. We lived in a kind of empty trance and each new session of the Seminar gave us the feeling that there was no way of finding a road into the Seminar itself.

Suddenly, in December 1975, a glimmer of light came peeping through. Lacan had just got back from the US and was speaking about Chomsky (Lacan, 2005a, pp. 27–43). We were acquainted with Chomsky. We had been able to take advantage of the lessons of Jean-Claude Milner, who was and has long remained the leading French Chomskyan. We thought, therefore, that we might find something here, some point of support. Next, in February 1976, a lesson of the Seminar ended with the following declaration: "Mad […]? […] this is not a privilege, […] in most people the symbolic, the imaginary and the real are tangled up […]." (Lacan, 2005a, p. 87)

We were starting to understand. For some of his audience a door was opening: we were hearing the flipside to "On a question prior to any possible treatment of psychosis" (Lacan, 2006, pp. 445–458). What had been established, or so we believed, as a radical distinction between madness as a result of *foreclosure*, and that which is not affected by foreclosure, was now being displaced. Between neurosis and psychosis, which hitherto stood apart like two distinct continents, there emerged a passage of generalisation. We didn't understand everything, but an altogether different world was fanning out for us, which we were just starting to glimpse. Likewise, the knots looked to be a theoretical instrument that was highly abstract (a long way from where we were standing) and yet clinical and pragmatic. The many indications about rectifying the "slipped knot" by means of the *sinthome* lay in this direction.

Amongst these indications, the discussion on Joyce's Catholicism that followed the lecture which you, Jacques Aubert, delivered in March 1976, holds an important place (Lacan, 1977a, pp. 16–17). Jacques-Alain Miller, Philippe Sollers and yourself each spoke on that occasion, and by way of reply Lacan gave some utterly fresh clinical indications. This was an *instant of seeing*. The building of Joyce's *Ego* revisits what features in "On a question prior to any possible treatment ..." in terms of an imaginary prosthesis. Starting off from the *sinthome*, this building of the *Ego* allows one to take up the writing of the "slipped knot".

What you have shared with us this evening[2] develops this question of the building of the *Ego* and allows us better to understand Lacan's indication concerning Joyce's "duplicated imaginary" (Lacan, 1977a, pp. 16–17).

At the time, this clinical indication given at the conference was crucial. Whereas the indications given in the Seminar on the duplication of the symbolic and the symptom were open to a good many readings, his indication of a "duplicated imaginary" that produces an "imaginary of security" offered a pragmatic translation of this duplication. In the wake of this *instant of seeing* there followed a lengthy *time for understanding* in which we still find ourselves today, thirty years on, but clearly this was the moment when our eyes were first opened. In November 1976, the clinical section got underway. The adventure of the clinical section was the time for understanding the indications that emanated from this point, from this flipside of the 1958 "Question".

An incandescent clinic

This clinical enquiry allowed Jacques-Alain Miller to differentiate carefully between the first and second clinics of Lacan. The first was focused on the Name-of-the-Father and its modalities whilst the second encompasses both the pluralisation of the Name-of-the-Father and, above all, the fact of language taking charge of jouissance. In the second clinic, the common nouns take charge of jouissance. What you have shared with us this evening, Jacques Aubert, clarifies the clinical perspectives that need to be used to show the point of passage from proper name to common noun, via the pluralisation of proper names. I shall take up your formulation on the neologistic use of *Nego*:

> I draw your attention to the fact that the passage from *nego*, with a lower case "n", to *Nego* with an upper case, is very clearly the passage not only from the space of the letter to the space of the name (which is not merely the space of the proper name), but specifically to a space for the *act* of naming.

This act, here associated with writing, both duplicates and shifts in a decisive way the value and weight of the *Ego*, which, after all, is a pronoun, that is, something that by definition comes to the place of the name. There is a "duplicated pronomination". Duplication is introduced between the *Ego* and its new symptomatic name, *Nego*. This duplication forms the matrix of the pluralisation of the new nouns that can be introduced into the common language, into the language of the master.

> It is clear that the fact that there are two names that are proper to the subject was an invention that spread as the story unfolded. That Joyce was also called James links up in a succession only with the use of the alias: James Joyce *also known as* Dedalus. The fact that we can pile up a whole stack of them ultimately leads to one thing: it introduces the proper name into the essence of the common noun.

Nego is …

Jacques Aubert: … Joyce's first neologism.

Éric Laurent: What the psychiatric clinic has termed "neologism" may be approached as a particular use of nouns. We may read the neologism as a word that belongs to the symptomatic languages that psychotics invent. Replacing *Ego* by *Nego* makes a negation appear in the place of the ego. More precisely, this substitution forms a hole. This way of hollowing out language, this introduction of an empty place, is distinct from the way in which Aristotle introduced the function of the place in his logical arguments by introducing letters.

The possibility of "place" was introduced into philosophical language on the basis of the Aristotelian syllogism. Starting off from this basis, one can deduce that if all men are mortal, and Socrates is a man, then Socrates is mortal. Socrates can be replaced by a letter and can be missing from his place.

Jacques Aubert has let us see how the common signification of a language can be found in a different way. It can even become entirely formed of holes, formed of new words or new ways of using common words. It may be said that at the end of *Finnegans Wake*, each word is a letter that is taken up in highly singularised networks. The Joyceans have to draw on their full gamut of knowledge to reconstruct them and to share them with us. This is why we go on reading your editions of Joyce.

The hole-less body and modular organs

Before I come back to this point, I would like first of all to take a detour via what Lacan introduced in December 1975 when he said the following about Chomsky:

> Dealing as he does with linguistics, I might have hoped to see in Chomsky some slither of appreciation of what I have been showing with respect to the symbolic, that is, that it maintains something of the hole [...].
>
> It is impossible, for instance, not to qualify the set formed by the symptom and the symbolic as a false hole. However [...] the symptom subsists in so far as it is hooked onto language [...].
>
> That Chomsky should assimilate to the real something that in my eyes belongs to the realm of the symptom, that is, that he should mix up the symptom and the real, is very precisely what took me aback. (Lacan, 2005a, p. 39)

That was back in 1975. Chomsky's programme was still blithe. He still thought that he could sustain his programme, given a few tweaks. For Chomsky at that time, mixing up the symptom and the real amounted to declaring that language is an organ. This was how Chomsky himself came to mend what was thwarted in the Artificial Intelligence programme.

We can consider this cognitive programme to have got underway—although this is a somewhat arbitrary start-point—with Gödel's theorem. In 1932, Gödel replied to a mathematical problem that David Hilbert had voiced some fifty years hence. The problem that Hilbert posed runs as follows: given any mathematical proposition, can a way be found to decide whether it is true or false? This problem is known as the *Entscheidungproblem*, the "decision problem". Gödel demonstrated, fifty years later, that this couldn't be done. You don't need to be dealing with a particularly complex system, as in arithmetic, to meet propositions that cannot be qualified either as true or as false. For this, Gödel invented a method that consisted not only in taking arithmetic statements as such (coding), but also in reducing any statement produced in the system to the form of a sequence of numerical figures.

This is what Alan Turing developed four years later, in 1936. He published the first article to perfect a logical "universal machine" (Turing,

1937), the same that thereafter bore his name. The "universal machine" enables any mathematical function to be defined on the basis of its calculability by the machine. This was achieved in concordance with the recursive functions that had been established by the logician Alonzo Church.

From this there emerged a current of thinkers who wanted to reduce all language, including the natural languages, to a mode of calculus. They thought it should be possible to show that speaking is a form of calculus and that a language stems from systems of calculus in general. This was the Artificial Intelligence research programme. Moreover, Herbert Simon, who was associated with this project, wrote a book with the fine title, *The Sciences of the Artificial* (Simon, 1969). For Simon, the artificial, the artefact, is reduced to a calculation that one should be able to turn into a science. The results obtained during the Second World War on the decipherment of encrypted messages gave encouragement to this perspective. Thereafter, however, they noticed that it was impossible to establish regularities in a language that would allow all the oddities of natural languages to be reduced to a calculation.

The limitations of this programme first started to appear in the 1950s, and this was when Chomsky put forward a programme that took off from a different standpoint. He wanted to develop a transformational model of the mind's cognitive capacities, conceived of in terms of information processing rather than logico-mathematical calculus. This information processing stems in part, but only in part, from logic and mathematics, from syntax transformation rules. It also had to be articulated with the laws of the living organism. This is the processing of information that has come from the living organism, or the living being treated as information. In a stroke of genius, Chomsky rewrote the existing structural grammars of the natural languages. He turned them into particular cases of rigorous rules of transformation that fall into the logico-mathematical category. So it was that he tried to obtain a universal grammar founded on these rules. At first, he enjoyed considerable success on the path of this universal grammar, or "language of thought" (LOT). This led him, along with his student Jerry Fodor, to specify what he understood by LOT-processing "modules". The evolution from the broad conception of language-calculus to the module that defines the specific task of a part of the mind is particularly clear in Fodor's work.

After writing *The Language of Thought* in 1975, Fodor published *The Modularity of Mind* in 1983. This latter book teases out the consequences of the work of an English psychologist, David Marr, whose findings on vision had been published posthumously in 1982. Marr set himself three distinct objectives. He argued that one has to determine: (i) the task of the visual system, that is, the computational transformation that it carries out; (ii) the algorithm that it implements in order to do so; and (iii) the manner in which this algorithm is materially realised in cerebral tissue (Marr, 1982, pp. 24–25).

This led to what Jean-Claude Milner called "Chomsky's sophisticated theory". More precisely, Milner underlined the new definition of the organ that this fresh approach entails:

> A good illustration of the sophisticated theory is met in David Marr (1982): according to the traditional conception, which is accepted as much in public opinion as it is in philosophy or in science, the organ of vision is none other than the eye, and, inversely, the best definition of the eye is to make it the organ of vision.
>
> Now, in Marr's theory, the organ is not the eye but the full set of interdependent anatomical devices that allow a reply to be given to the question "what is where?" These devices are numerous and heterogeneous. Each of them contributes in modular fashion to articulate one of the elements of the pertinent response. In other words, the somatic approach only attains a dispersed multiplicity; the definitory unit of the organ can only be obtained in functional terms, the question "what is where?" (which Marr lifts explicitly from Aristotle) being merely a roundabout way of defining the visual function. The visual organ as such can only be specified in relation to this function. It has no other unity but this. One may consider the word "vision" to designate, somewhat ambiguously, both the organ, O (and in this sense vision is strictly speaking an organ) and the function, F. Thereafter, the material unity that the eye seemed to constitute is reduced to sheer appearance: this material unity may be compromised, but still the actual unity of the visual organ will not be called into question. (Milner, 1989, p. 207)

The new paradigm of cognition thus defines a pluralisation of modules that give rise to a whole host of new organs housed in a body in which they proliferate. In 1975, when Lacan was returning from the US, Chomsky still thought that he was dealing with one organ. From 1980 onwards, there was a multiplication of organs, they were abounding. This gave us a body covered in organs, covered in modules. These organs function in an almost autistic way, leading Fodor to declare that the current state of affairs is tantamount to a modularity "gone mad" (Fodor, 1987, p. 27).

Jean-Claude Milner considers that in spite of this excess the fact of having grasped language on the basis of cognitive modules that respond to precise questions of the "what is where?" sort, (rather than on the basis of a law, of the universal syntax sort) allows precise forms of knowledge to be defined. This paradigm allows for a modelisation of certain phenomena of language that the generative-transformational system did not manage to tackle, especially one particular phenomenon that has been close to Milner's heart for a long time: questions of *anaphor*. This is where we meet up with Jacques Aubert and the particular anaphor he has just presented.

Pronominalisation is one way for the subject to make a hole in language at several different sites using pronouns, using proper names, using their conveyance and the way they create holes in a statement. This was how Jean-Claude Milner gave serious consideration to Lacan's indications in *Le sinthome*. It was precisely a matter not of reducing language to an organ but of ascertaining how holes are made in a language. On this point, Milner has set out reflections of such precision and quality that I can only urge you to refer to his work.

The new definitions of the cognitive paradigm or the cognitive "venture" leave these questions open. The great advantage of Chomsky—which is appearing now in our debates and struggles with the cognitive-behavioural therapies—is that his idea of the language-organ shattered all the behaviourist ideas. It shattered any possibility of speech as a learning process in a body bereft of language. Behaviourism tended to consider that the subject only learns to speak through imitation, followed by reinforcement and aversion. In the behaviourist view, the subject was dealing with a mute body that was then conditioned. The idea of the language-organ, of language that is both organ and algorithm, as it were, constitutes a radical objection to this. This organ is something living that has already been caught up in a language that was there beforehand.

The sack and its detachable organs

Lacan's Seminar on *Le sinthome* expresses his eagerness to articulate language with the living being on the basis of the hole. On one side lies

Chomsky's path, which was to lead to the proliferation of organs, and on the other side lies Lacan's. Lacan was to link up the organ-less body, the body of the empty set, the body as a sack, with the consistency of the cords of language that traverse it around a hole.

He was to put forward "a rope-and-sack logic", as Jacques-Alain Miller has underscored.[3] The ropes are there to tie a knot in the sack, to link it up with the hole. Rather than indicating the consistency of the knot in the form of a ring, he presents it in the form of the infinite straight line, thereby avoiding any imaginary aspect of a circle that encloses.

In particular, says Lacan, a circle is evocative of all kinds of parasitic things, most especially the delimitations of nerve centres (Lacan, 2005a, p. 145). What we call "nerve centres", neuronal localisations on the cortex, are always the result of an attempt—and nowadays this is done with ever more modern instruments such as tomographic cameras or magnetic resonance imaging—to concretise the hope of reducing signification to a circle. In actual fact, what one discovers in these increasingly advanced procedures in the study of the nervous system are interconnections that simply go on and on. Each region stands in relation to a number of further regions, and so the organs come to be defined more with respect to modular considerations.

So, on one side there is the Joyce/Lacan pole, on the other the Chomsky pole. For Lacan, the body is not kitted out with these strange, modularised organs, it is kitted out with the *sinthome*. This is what has consistency, even though it is articulated with the hole in the symbolic. Lacan asserts this by means of the cord, and he adds that what strikes him as absolutely necessary when it comes to defining the very idea of language is that language is what empties out the real, it "eats into the real".

> Indeed, to my mind, if one doesn't admit the principial truth that language is tied to something that makes a hole in the real, it is not simply difficult, but impossible to consider how it is handled. Observational method cannot start off from language without it emerging that the latter makes a hole in what can be situated as real. It is on the basis of this function of the hole that language effectuates its purchase on the real. (Lacan, 2005a, p. 31)

Lacan qualifies the relationship between the body and the organs as "detachable". He borrows an example from an anthropologist who showed that a flying bullet is not the extension of the arm but a detachment of the arm, the arm projected (Lacan, 2005a, p. 86). For Lacan, the organs are thus detachable:

> The *parlêtre* adores his body because he believes that he has it. In reality, he doesn't, but his body is his only consistency—his only mental consistency, you understand—because his body will bugger off at any moment. (Lacan, 2005a, p. 66)

This point of view is utterly distinct from Freud's in *Civilisation and its Discontents*, which sets out a body whose organs are its extension:

> With every tool man is perfecting his own organs, whether motor or sensory, or is removing the limits to their functioning. Motor power places gigantic forces at his disposal, which, like his muscles, he can employ in any direction; thanks to ships and aircraft neither water nor air can hinder his movements; by means of spectacles he corrects defects in the lens of his own eye; by means of the telescope he sees into the far distance; and by means of the microscope he overcomes the limits of visibility set by the structure of his retina. In the photographic camera he has created an instrument which retains the fleeting visual impressions, just as a gramophone disc retains the equally fleeting auditory ones; both are at bottom materialisations of the power he possesses of recollection, his memory. With the help of the telephone he can hear at distances which would be respected as unattainable even in a fairly tale. Writing was in its origin the voice of an absent person; and the dwelling-house was a substitute for the mother's womb, the first lodging, for which in all likelihood man still longs, and in which he was safe and felt at ease. (Freud, 1930a, pp. 89–90)

The real is thus also presented with the same meaning that Lacan gave to it in 1974 in an interview for the Italian magazine *Panorama*: the real has replaced nature, and the real is advancing (Lacan, 1974). This real is composed through scientific discourse. It is made up of objects that have nothing natural about them. It is formed of ways of proceeding, of procedures. The real advances, just as Nietzsche said that the desert advances.[4] It lies radically beyond meaning, but language allows us to fasten onto it by producing "enjoy-meant". It is not a question of giving meaning to this real. The question of the modern subject is not a "loss of meaning", as Hillary Clinton would say.[5] It is not a matter of slapping on any extra, but of allowing the letter to stand a chance of operating in language, to stand a chance of forming holes of equivocation, to stand a chance of managing to break up the universalised signifiers that bear down upon us without having the faintest relationship with us.

These objects in which our desire is enclosed, which pass over to the condition of being the "cause of desire", still have to be appropriated between the lines. For Lacan, language was indeed to be defined as a sort of organ, but a symptom-organ. The object *a*, as a lamella, is an organ (Lacan, 2006, p. 718). As an organ, the object *a* covers the body and plugs up all of its orifices. The body plugged by the object *a* is the true organ-less body. With language, one manages to form orifices, one manages to have oral, anal, scopic and invocatory orifices; that is, one manages to form a rim for each of these orifices.

In early-onset psychosis, in autism, one can observe just what a rim-less organ is, and also the heroic attempts these subjects make to create a rim. The object *a* could be represented as a bubble-gum balloon: it is what allows for the creation of a breathing space that doesn't collapse back onto your mouth and doesn't splatter over your whole body when it bursts. The same goes for all the body's rims.

Lacan's "rope-and-sack" logic is a logic that is articulated between, on one hand, the sack that could find itself completely plugged up by the real, and on the other, the rope that allows for a way through and for these rims and orifices to be constructed. Thus, the body's true consistency is not the consistency of the sack but the consistency of the rope, the cord. This assumes that the subject does not ground his identification, his seat in the world, on the basis of his swelling form, his bodily envelope, the narcissism of the image, but that he manages to get by in constituting drive-circuits, the drifting trajectory of the drive, *sinthomatically*.

Image fetishism

Joyce is the one who manages to create a drifting trajectory of the drive. He slides. *Finnegans Wake* is a dream where the dreamer is nowhere. He is the dream itself. We are confronted with nouns of a tongue that become proper names. These are the names of the dreamer himself. Finnegan is consubstantial with them and these proper names become the common names of the idiosyncratic tongue that it is up to us to decipher. Lacan says, "It is in this respect that Joyce slides and slides and slides, to Jung, and to the collective unconscious" (Lacan, 2005a, p. 125). Psychoanalysis implies guiding him onto that drifting trajectory of the drive in which something of the dreamer can still be assigned. The dreamer is then assigned a place by the traces of jouissance that animate the dream as a whole.

Although we isolate two polarities (Joyce and Chomsky) in the relationships to the language-organ, at the end of the day we have to find our own specific language-organ, our language-organ of the *sinthome*, which effectively poses an obstacle to any totalising conception of the image. Now, the functioning of civilisation is thrown together in such a way that it favours in every aspect identification with the totalising image; hence the publicity industry, hence "commodity fetishism", to use Marx's excellent term that arose from the shock he felt on visiting the Great Exhibition of 1851.

The first time that Marx saw all those industrial products lined up at the Exhibition in the vast buildings of London's Crystal Palace, he identified this commodity fetishism. We've gone much further today. Not a single shop can refrain from capturing the browser in ideal bodies with which he is beckoned to identify and which are covered in fantasmatic accessories that fasten onto him or strive to do so. As Lacan put it in the aforementioned interview: "this rampant sexomania is just a publicity phenomenon" (Lacan, 1974).

The cognition of the therapy that has been termed "cognitive-behavioural" has nothing to do with the cognitive programme and everything to do with this belief that people have in their image. The cognition of the cognitive-behavioural therapies consists, as it has done since their invention back in the late 1950s, in identifying with an ideal image.

The cognitive-behavioural therapy of depression devised by Aaron Beck (a former psychoanalyst who changed tack in search of rapid efficacy) consists in persuading the subject that he has a systematic negative-judgement bias towards his own person. The subject's life story has to be worked over so that it will allow for something positive to be established. This positive bias has to be systematically pitted against the negative bias. They call this "cognitive reframing". It is a matter of identifying the subject with a successful image of himself. If it is done sufficiently—and the term "reframing" is absolutely the right one—the subject will become locked onto a different image of himself. The subject is offered a different window and a different image. This is the therapy's point of leverage. It is a matter of making the subject believe in this positive image of himself.

Albert Bandura's therapy for violent children, which lies at the origin of another style of CBT, consists in offering such children models of calm. They have to be turned away from violent models and placed in different environments. From this, Bandura deduced a much wider political project. He wanted to make violence vanish altogether from television and cinema. Forty years on, we can see what a failure this has been. Social hygiene movements seem to have been particularly powerless in this respect. Violence has pervaded everything. The hidden logic of this is the jouissance behind each blow levelled at the ideal image in all its forms, and indeed this passion is commensurate with the fetishism of the image.

Science fiction

The subject's belief in the soul, such as it is defined in *Le sinthome*, is the ineradicable residue of the bodily image (Lacan, 2005a, p. 150). The soul leads us by the nose. We have an excellent example of this in the therapeutic approach that consists in immersing the subject in video games that have been transformed into a cognitive learning procedure. He no longer needs a therapist; the machine itself is enough to work its suggestion on the user. On one hand, the power of the ideal image dispenses with any reference to the body of the other party and his presence; on the other, the body's autism is commandeered by the machine.

In a recent study carried out by the National Institute for Health and Care Excellence (NICE) in the UK, the widespread use of therapies without therapists was put to the test. It assessed computerised cognitive-behaviour therapy (CCBT) for the treatment of anxiety, depression, phobias, panic attacks and other forms of OCD. It is also specified that this research includes CCBT by internet. I shall simply cite two recommendations that NICE gave for any future research (Kaltenthaler et al., 2002, p. 77):

> Research is needed to compare CCBT to other therapies that reduce therapist time, in particular bibliotherapy.
>
> [...]
>
> Studies of CCBT should be randomised controlled trials and need to include an intention-to-treat (ITT) analysis in order to

take into account patients who drop out of trials. The reasons for withdrawal from trials need to be identified as this relates directly to patient preference.

Indeed, one ought never to forget just to what extent CBT statistics fail to indicate how they select the subjects they adopt. The only subjects who remain in these testing-procedures are those that can put up with them. This is where the *universal* right to these therapies meets the *particular*. As Jean Cottraux puts it:

> Behavioural therapy was behind substantial and lasting improvements in 50–70% of sufferers who took part in the full set of planned sessions. Limits did appear, however. According to the more pessimistic statistics, 25% of patients who presented an indication of behavioural therapy refused to undergo it. Out of the remaining 75%, 25% did not improve. Out of the 50% who improved, 20% relapsed in the space of between three months and three years. These figures compel therapeutic modesty and invite further research into new forms of treatment, both biological and psychological.

These are the words of a master in the field, and we should never forget just how often these authoritarian therapies turn off a number of those who undergo them. Indeed, therapies such as these ultimately give rise to a de-segregative desire.

This desire is what allows us to keep open the path of the symptom, articulated around language. And this is precisely where the subject dwells, the subject as a response from the real.

Notes

1. Lacan's 1975–6 Seminar, *Le sinthome*, established as *Livre XXIII* by Jacques-Alain Miller, was published by Éditions du Seuil in March 2005.
2. Published as Aubert, 2005. A later, more developed, version of this paper was published in English as Aubert, 2010.
3. Cf., the subheadings to Chapter X of Lacan, 2005a, p. 143.
4. Cf., Nietzsche, F., *Dithyrambs of Dionysus*.
5. Hillary Clinton quoted in Sheely, 1999, p. 173. See also Clinton, 2003, pp. 160–1: "We need a new politics of meaning" (from her 6 April 1993 speech on health).

CHAPTER TWO

Neural plasticity and the impossible inscription of the subject

The Freudian unconscious has now found a translation in the language of the neurosciences. This at least is the new paradigm that the supporters of cognitive psychoanalysis have been attempting to establish across the entirety of the field in the wake of Eric Kandel's work.

Kandel wanted to make psychoanalysis shift from its pre-scientific "context of discovery" to a higher scientific level by absorbing it into the new discipline of cognitive neuroscience (Kandel, 1999, p. 506). This project took shape in two famous articles that preceded his Nobel Prize in Medicine, which was awarded for his work on memory storage. Kandel's project is a radical one and he has been seeking to convince all psychoanalysts of its legitimacy.

Kandel's neurological work concerns memory in general and its patterns of inscription in the nervous system. Having been interested in psychoanalysis as a young doctor (he was an acquaintance of the family of the famous analyst Ernst Kris) he opted to study the memory of learning and its traces in the brain, "one cell at a time" (Kandel, 2006, pp. 53–73). He studied the changes in synaptic exchanges produced by traditional conditioned-learning procedures.

In 1970 Eric Kandel and his team highlighted the functional changes of synapses in aplysia correlative with learning processes. [...] [Three years later] in their initial discovery [Timothy Bliss & Terje Lømo] showed that [in rabbits] a short high-frequency stimulation of a neuronal pathway that transmits sensory information from the cortex to the hippocampus induces a considerable and lasting increase in the efficacy of synaptic transmission: the target neurons in the hippocampus acquire greater sensitivity with each successive stimulus. The most remarkable aspect of this form of plasticity, which is induced in the tenth of a millisecond, is its persistence: the synapses remain in their modified state for weeks, even for months. This discovery gave rise to great enthusiasm in the scientific community. Could this be, they wondered, the mechanism for memory storage in the brain [...]? (Laroche, 2001)[1]

The repetitive procedures of this form of memory call upon neither consciousness nor the language that presupposes a subject. They are conceived of as a module that employs various systems: the motor-sensory cortex, the amygdalae, the hippocampus, and so on. The experiential inscription model that Kandel puts forward acknowledges its sources in Pavlov, but he generalises Pavlov by drafting in the notion of contingent association that Leon Kamin proposed in 1969 (Kamin, 1969). The nervous system's capacity to be modified by experience defines its plasticity.

This can give rise to standard, mechanistic interpretations. Take for example the interpretation proposed by the recipient of a prize from the French Association of Biological Psychiatry at the seventh colloquium of the Société des neurosciences:

The notion of "neuro-plasticity" designates the capacity of neurones to modify their molecular structure and interconnections over the course of a lifetime. Closely linked to neuro-genesis and apoptosis, neuro-plasticity regulates the brain's interactions with its environment, its history and its genome. The discovery of neuro-genesis in 1998 overturned a dogma: the adult human brain is well and truly capable of producing new cells, in particular at the level of the hippocampus, a structure that is indispensable for memory. Recurrent depression would seem to be characterised by a lowering in the synthesis of growth factors, hence lower neuro-plasticity and an imbalance between neuro-genesis and apoptosis. These phenomena would seem to accompany recurrently depressed individuals and lie at the origin of a progressive atrophy of the hippocampus, the morphological substrate of the episodic memory disturbances observed in recurrent depressed patients. (Radtchenko, 2005)

In the next passage we can see how, for this author, neuronal plasticity merely extends the realm of the mental automaton by opening the door to further hypotheses, and even to new treatments that use electrical or chemical stimulation:

The stress that is implicit in depression would seem to have a harmful effect on the hippocampus due to a prolonged production of excitotoxic corticosteroids and amino acids. The hippocampus, equipped as it is with serotonin receptors, would be one of the main targets of anti-depressant agents. Atrophy of the hippocampus in animals would seem to be partially reversible with prolonged action of anti-depressants by virtue of stimulating neuro-plasticity. (Radtchenko, 2005)

Kandel on the other hand offers a reading of behavioural memory (types of behaviour that bypass consciousness) in terms of the Freudian hypothesis of unconscious processes. This leads him to coin the term "procedural unconscious". By the same stroke, the Freudian notion of anxiety as a signal faced with a trauma seems to him to be explained perfectly by Pavlov, whilst the role of the amygdalae in regulating anxiety allows him to give an account of the treatment of post-traumatic anxiety.

For Kandel, the crux of what happens in psychoanalysis takes place at the level of processes of repetition and "changes in behaviour that increase the patient's range of procedural strategies for doing and being". Thus, it takes place outside the dimension of interpretation and outside the dimension of meaning. Those few moments when the procedural unconscious might be accessible to consciousness, or to meaning (the two terms are interchangeable in Kandel), hold little importance (Kandel, 1999, p. 509).

This translation in terms of the neuronal network of subjective processes *qua* memory processing is strongly disputed by other voices from the neurosciences who oppose this conception of memory as storage. For example, Bennett and Hacker:

> It is very tempting to think that the diverse forms in which remembering something may be manifest are all due to the fact that what is remembered is *recorded* and *stored* in the brain. But that is a nonsense. *What is remembered* when it is remembered that such-and-such is not anything laid down in the brain […], but rather something previously learnt or experienced. What neuroscientists must try to discover is what are the neural conditions of remembering and the neural concomitants of recollecting something […]
>
> The expression of a memory must be distinguished from the neural configurations, whatever they may be, which are conditions for a person's recollecting whatever he recollects. But these configurations are not memory; nor are they representations, depictions or expressions of what is remembered. (Bennet & Hacker, 2003, p. 170)

The act of remembering cannot be reduced to some norm of accessing a stored memory that is more or less immutable in its forms, any change in which would be explained away by some sort of entropic erosion. This kind of unconscious memory of the body and its acts may be entertained for the routines to which the body yields without paying further attention. It might be suitable for a wide variety of habitual actions and a broad range of practices, for anything indeed that falls in the "learning" category. But it is not suitable for all that corresponds to a subjective act, to all that constitutes an event, which when it does happen happens but once (*alea iacta est*), and which is felt in the body in the form of a very different trace. This is why other theoretical solutions have not failed to make themselves heard.

Somato-psychical plasticity

Pierre Magistretti and François Ansermet have offered a solution by which to articulate the neurosciences and psychoanalysis which is distinct from Kandel's model. In a book first published in 2004, they take on board Kandel's accepted notion of "psychical trace", but in so doing accentuate plasticity rather than the trace itself. They start by comparing Kandel's trace with the Freudian trace:

> Perception can leave a trace in the nervous system and become memory. In other words, perception leaves a sign inscribed in the neural circuits, one that could be identified with the Freudian concept of the sign of perception. (Ansermet & Magistretti, 2007, p. 18)

In a more recent article the authors reconsider this conception as just one experimental model amongst others:

> These phenomena are at the basis of the processes of learning and memory. One of the experimental models which have been largely studied is long-term potentiation which can modify the efficacy of synaptic transfer. (Ansermet & Magistretti, 2008, p. 475)

The essential component is plasticity:

> This observation has found experimental confirmation through recent progress in neurobiology, which demonstrates a plasticity of the neuronal network permitting the inscription of experience. (Ansermet & Magistretti, 2007, p. xiii)

They call into question the notion of a brain reduced to a pure automaton of traces by considering not only inscription in the cortex but in the body too: the somato-psychical bond.

> The second major argument we shall be setting forth in this book is that the constitution of this unconscious internal reality based on the mechanisms of plasticity is not exclusively a mental phenomenon but involves the body as well. For we shall be discussing the fact that the traces left by experience are associated with somatic traces. Our argument is that the perceptions leaving a trace in the synaptic network are associated with a somatic state.
>
> This claim is based on a whole set of recent data in the neurobiological literature, synthesised by Antonio Damasio (1994) in the theory of somatic markers. (Ansermet & Magistretti, 2007, pp. xvii–xviii)

Their conception of plasticity allows them to avoid the negative criticism that Damasio's conception has drawn. The main criticism concerns the fixed correspondence that Damasio sets out between a bodily state and an emotion. This criticism has been expressed in different ways. One of the first came from Bennett and Hacker:

> Damasio [...] distinguishes *an emotion* [...] from the *feeling of an emotion*. [...] An emotion is a bodily response to a mental image, and the feeling of an emotion is a cognitive response to the bodily condition [...]. Feelings of emotion, Damasio avers, "are just *as cognitive as any other perceptual image*, and just as dependent on cerebral-cortex processing as any other image." (Bennet & Hacker, 2003, pp. 210–212)

So, from this perspective the vocabulary for the emotive and affective register is, in his final analysis, none other than the precise emotion that is felt in the body. He holds that it is possible to establish a one-to-one mapping of *feelings* in relation to states of the body (*emotions*).

Ian Hacking offers a different formulation of the critique of fixity, concluding that within this perspective there is no more subject, there are merely "homeostatic" states:

> Feelings and emotions have been part of the language of persons, both for expressing my self and for describing others. Damasio proposes something different: instant anatomical identification of emotions; this is what they really *are*, that is what joy *is*. [...] [T]here seems in Damasio's account to be no "I" left who decides how to handle [any given] situation. (Hacking, 2004a, pp. 35–36)

There is no more metaphorical or metonymical sliding possible, despite the fact that the register of affects is part and parcel of language. Fixity is reinforced by this conception of emotion as a somatic marker to be regulated.

> [According to Damasio] "Emotions play out in the theatre of the body. Feelings play out in the theatre of the mind." Both are *for* [...] "life regulation" but feelings do it at a higher level. Joy is the feeling of life in equilibrium; sorrow of life in disarray ("functional disequilibrium"). [...]
>
> Both feelings and emotions are states, conditions or processes in the body. An emotion such as pity "is a complex collection of

chemical and neural responses forming a distinctive pattern."
(Hacking, 2004a, pp. 32–33)

Damasio's conception is one of an organism without any Other; an organism that is profoundly autistic, folded in upon homeostatic auto-regulation that is perfected through the course of evolution.

In their later article, Ansermet and Magistretti complexify the relationships between the synaptic trace and the body by retaining from Damasio's model only the necessity for homeostasis, which they subject to a profound transformation by linking it to the Freudian pleasure principle. The trace is not only the effect of the organism's experience of meeting the outside, it comes from the body's inside too (which is also "in exteriority" with respect to the system of traces), to the extent that, as the authors argue, the brain acts upon the body in order to maintain homeostasis.

> As a general point, one can say that the maintenance of homeostasis is a central feature of any living organism as was postulated by Claude Bernard, with the concept of the constancy of the "internal milieu". One can say that the brain is in a way the supreme organ for the maintenance of homeostasis. [...]
>
> The homeostatic requirement thus situates the organism outside the subject, along with the reality in which he is immersed. This view, therefore, suggests that the mental reality of the subject is not simply constituted by traces in direct relationship with perception. A discontinuity exists whereby traces are linked to somatic states, and through their associations and re-arrangements, depending on the homeostatic requirement and in relation to the actions of the subject, they produce a discontinuity which goes well beyond the simple inscription of experience [...].
>
> [...]
>
> A central place should therefore be given to the biology of the interoceptive system which permanently informs the brain of the somatic states. (Ansermet & Magistretti, 2008, pp. 476–477)[2]

In maintaining this requirement to go beyond the "simple inscription of experience", the authors are able to affirm that it must be possible to follow the path that leads from experience to the inscription of subjectivity.

[...] one can say that it is possible to follow how perception is inscribed under the form of traces and consider how traces become associated between them later on. One can also consider the biological basis of the somatic markers. The integration of these different levels should be at the centre of the questions posed to attempt an understanding of mental phenomena. (Ansermet & Magistretti, 2008, p. 477)

They underline, however, that psychical phenomena as such consist in the discontinuity between inscription and behaviour.

[...] there is not a simple and direct mapping of a stimulus, its perception and its inscription in the neuronal network. In the same way, there is not a simple mapping between these inscriptions and the behaviour which will result from it. One should think in terms of discontinuity between the stimulus, its inscription and the response produced by the subject if one wants to understand what a mental phenomenon is. [...] The notion of neuronal plasticity produces a series of paradoxes which re-introduce the notion of the subject in biology. (Ansermet & Magistretti, 2008, p. 477)

Thus the authors share Bennett and Hacker's refusal to consider the experience of memory in relation to the storing of traces of experience. The freshness of their conception and the paradoxes they highlight allow us to perceive just how often, in any complex experience, the relation between the trace that is inscribed and the event that provoked it is very rapidly broken off. Far from ensuring a correspondence, the system of traces tends rather to inscribe the *loss* of any correspondence between the trace and the initial experience.

From trace to trace, from inscription to re-inscription to the re-association of traces, the link and connection between the initial experience and the traces is somehow lost, even though the initial traces maintain a direct link with experience. Thus, plasticity introduces a discontinuity. [...]

As a general point, one could say that as far as the establishment of the unconscious is concerned, inscription of experience separates from experience. The unconscious is therefore not a memory system. This point leads to a paradox in which memory in its relationship with the unconscious does not represent a means to preserve experience under the form of traces of perception. (Ansermet & Magistretti, 2008, p. 477)

The lessons that the authors draw from this non-preservation of experience on the basis of traces are twofold. On one hand, this non-preservation constitutes the foundation of the inscription of the singularity of each subject's experience when faced with an internal or external stimulus.

> Through the unique interplay mediated by the re-association of traces, the universal mechanisms of plasticity result in the production of a unique subject, each time different. One could say that in this way and paradoxically plasticity implies a determination of the unpredictable.
>
> Neuronal plasticity modifies neuronal networks; thus two stimuli, even though identical, could result in different responses depending on the state of the brain. As in a game of chess, everything depends on the move that has been made previously. Plasticity introduces a variability which removes any idea of an equal, univocal and determined response through a system which would be rigid and fixed in time. One never uses the same brain twice! (Ansermet & Magistretti, 2008, p. 478)

Or further still:

> Plasticity entails the obvious fact that, through the sum of lived experiences, each individual is seen to be unique and unpredictable beyond the determinations of his genetic background. The universal laws defined by neurobiology thus inevitably end in the production of the unique. The question of the subject as an exception to the universal now becomes as central for the neurosciences as it is for psychoanalysis, leading to an unexpected meeting point between these two protagonists, so accustomed to being antagonists. (Ansermet & Magistretti, 2007, pp. 6–7)

On the other hand, the non-preservation of traced experience inscribes a fundamental indeterminacy into any possible inscription of experience. This is what the authors call, employing an oxymoron, a necessary "determination of the unpredictable" (Ansermet & Magistretti, 2008, p. 478).

> In the functioning of genes there are in fact mechanisms intended to leave room for experience, and these enter into play in the fulfilment of the genetic programme, as though, when all is said and done, the individual were to appear genetically determined not to be genetically determined. (Ansermet & Magistretti, 2007, p. 8)

Or further still:

> Plasticity thus enables us to take maximal advantage of the spectrum of possible differences, leaving due place to the unpredictable in the construction of individuality, and the individual can be considered to be biologically determined to be free, that is, to constitute an exception to the universal that carries him. (Ansermet & Magistretti, 2007, p. 10)

The authors read these two lessons as synonymous. We should like to urge them, however, not to consider them thus. On one hand, there is room for the renewal of the inscription of synapses and in this sense, indeed, one does not use the same brain twice, but on the other hand, there is the radical impossibility of reducing subjective inscription to a series of traces to the extent that the link between trace and experience is constantly being re-written.

It is precisely because the link with biological experience is lost that a non-biological identification, a signifying identification, can be produced. The language system functions as a supplementation to this hiatus. It is precisely because there is no biological memory that there can be a memory of the unconscious. It is in this respect that Lacan spoke not of a somatic/psychical cut (which would set apart body and psyche) but an epistemic/somatic cut. On one side lies that part of experience that is inscribed in the body, and on the other lies the knowledge that is set down on the basis of this experience. Biological discontinuity means that the subject fastens onto the signifier whose fastening to experience slips away. Rather than saying, as do our two authors, that we are "genetically programmed to be free", we might say that we are genetically programmed to be alienated from the signifier.

Inscription and discontinuity

It is through this very alienation that a point of passage emerges from the necessarily limited experiences of learning, or from each individual's experiences, to the infinite number of possible sentences that can describe such experiences. It is at this point that we meet the problem of the infinite potentiality of language, which has always posed a quandary for theories of experiential learning.

Chomsky had already levelled this objection at Skinner's behaviourist conception:

> [...] what does it mean to say that some sentence of English that I have never heard or produced belongs to my "repertoire", but not any sentence of Chinese (so that the former has a higher "probability")? Skinnerians, at this point in the discussion, appeal to "similarity" or "generalisation", but always without characterising precisely the ways in which a new sentence is "similar" to familiar examples or "generalised" from them. The reason for this failure is simple. So far as is known, the relevant properties can be expressed only by the use of abstract theories (for example, a grammar) describing postulated internal states of the organism, and such theories are excluded, a priori, from Skinner's "science". (Chomsky, 1971, p. 9)

This objection can also be formulated in the terms of Jean-Claude Milner:

> If everything in language is *acquired*, how might one explain that, on the basis of experiences that are necessarily finite in number and diversity, the subject is able to produce constructions that he has never met? This argument will have taken on an especially strong form when one adds that language is infinite, because the experiences that would allow for its acquisition are necessarily finite in number and limited in qualitative diversity. (Milner, 1989, p. 207)

Extending Chomsky's objection, Milner brings to light the paradox that is harboured in this phenomenon. The question of infinitude in language is Janus-faced. It is a property that is intrinsic to all languages, and yet it still has "no true empirical scope" for linguistics. Let's look with Milner at this first property:

> Knowing a language consists precisely in producing sentences that one has never heard. This possibility, which the Cambridge school has summed up with the term "competence", is beyond any doubt. More exactly, to research into its base is to research into the base of language itself, whether this base is understood as a transcendent source or as a material origin or as something else. In any case, the science of language only has conjectures to advance on this point and, in most of its versions, it takes the property of "infinitisation" for granted, even to the point of not fully realising that it has pre-supposed it: structural linguistics bears this out. Paradoxically, it therefore has to be admitted that the procedure of passing from the finite to potential infinitude, which remains problematic when the natural sciences are at issue, can be supposed to have been given as an objective property when language is at issue. By the same token, amplifying induction is always possible for the linguist: directly if he himself speaks the language he is studying; indirectly if he draws on an informant. (Milner, 1989, p. 636)

The role that this property plays, however, as fundamental as it may be for any possible linguistics, is not for all that particularly easy to specify.

> The potential existence of infinite sequences may be acknowledged: the fact is that it does not play any active role in syntax; such that the quarrel about linguistic infinitude, as lively as it has been, still has no true empirical scope. (Milner, 1989, p. 487)

We may say, following Milner, that the true scope of the question of linguistic infinitude, beyond the empirical, is to send us back to the discontinuity of cause, to the discontinuity that lies between, on one hand a subject's determination by contingency and by his experiences, and on the other what Kant called the subject's autonomy. Jacques-Alain Miller defines this discontinuity as follows:

> In a certain respect, the Kantian subject that we find in the *Critique of Practical Reason* is a loophole in objective causality, in

what is scientifically determinable. This subject cannot be directly perceived. One only meets Kant's famous categorical imperative, and only as a fact of the signifier. One runs aground on his formula. The formula is utterly inexplicable if one does not posit the existence of a suprasensible subject, a free subject that escapes from scientific causality. [...] Kant is the support we require to face up to the hegemony of scientific causality and the neurosciences, and to demonstrate that one can think about the subject in an entirely different dimension. Speaking about the autonomy of the subject means that the subject is barred in so far as he can be set apart from any objective conditioning. It is not a matter of saying, after this, that he is an autonomous subject, because he is dependent in his own specific dimension. It is a matter of accentuating the subject's dependence, but at a different level: at the level of the suprasensible, such as Kant defined it. (Miller, 2003a, pp. 28–29)

What is crucial here is the cut between the laws of language, which will have determined any "language-organ" regardless of its conception, and the possible inscription of the subject as an "automaton".

It is in this sense that we understand the "incommensurability" between the neurosciences and psychoanalysis by which Ansermet and Magistretti abide:

The incommensurability of these two fields, however, remains a stubborn fact. There is no syncretism between the neurosciences and psychoanalysis, no reconciliation, no possible synthesis. [...] These differences are a dynamic factor from which the emergence of the subject can be inferred, including on the basis of the laws of biology. (Ansermet & Magistretti, 2007, p. 11)

The epistemic/somatic cut and incommensurability

I propose, therefore, to lean on this "epistemic/somatic cut" between knowledge and inscription in the body in order to ground the incommensurability we have been speaking about. This cut must be preserved all the more given the great temptation to reduce subjective experience to a system of somatic traces.

This temptation may seem to be legitimised by discoveries of further biological systems that have been cropping up as candidates for the reception-site of the system of experiential traces. For example, criticism of an overly mechanistic conception of genetics has accentuated the importance of the "epigenetic imprint". One line of research has set out to explore just how far the subject's experiences will determine the way that genes find expression and become regulated:

> This is a way of modifying how easily a gene can be read.
>
> Moshe Szyf, of McGill University in Montreal, studies the effect of maternal care on epigenetic imprinting. As he explained at this week's meeting on Epigenetics and Neural Development Disorders, held in Beltsville, Maryland, imprinting might be a general mechanism whereby experiences are translated into behaviour. If that turns out to be so, it will affect understanding and treatment of mental illness. (*The Economist*, 2006b, pp. 78–79)

For the moment, the impact of epigenetic imprinting is limited to the first week of life after birth. This ambition to uncover the imprint system amounts to nothing less than a hope to account for highly complex conduct, such as suicidal and high-risk human behaviour, by searching for the same differential imprints in rats.

> [The] first human study is into whether those who commit suicide have different imprints in their hippocampuses from those who die in accidents. They are also studying blood samples from people with depression or with violent headaches, to look for epigenetic markers that may exist for either of these two behaviours. If successful, that might lead to new methods of diagnosing psychiatric conditions. (*The Economist*, 2006b, p. 79)

Meanwhile, elsewhere, linguists inspired by the neurosciences have also been seeking to form a conception of language and its metaphors as inscriptions. Following Chomsky, though less demanding than he when it comes to the precise nature of the organ of language, his former students like George Lakoff consider that it goes without saying to speak of linguistic structures as having been "fixed in the neural structures of [...] brains" by sheer repetition. Other linguists, however Darwinian they might be, worry about this uncritical habit of resorting to fixation in the brain:

It is true that "the frames that define common sense are instantiated in the brain", but only in the sense that every thought we think—permanent or transient, rational or irrational—is instantiated physically in the brain. [...] Cognitive psychology has not shown that people absorb frames through sheer repetition. On the contrary, information is retained when it fits into a person's greater understanding of the subject matter. Nor is the claim that people are locked into a single frame anywhere to be found in cognitive linguistics, which emphasises that people can nimbly switch among the many framings made available by their language. (Pinker, 2006)

The enchantment with thinking about any language or any experience as having been inscribed in the brain (or in a pattern of gene regulation) can give rise to the *furor sanandi* of neurosurgeons. Some of them are already entertaining the idea of making cerebral improvements, of "brain-lifts", which would be able to stimulate an ageing organ. In a recently published book, carefully setting aside any ethical dimension that such treatments would pose, one practitioner promotes the clear benefits of such cosmetic practices for their beneficiaries:

> Writing of a successful Manhattan neurosurgeon she knows whose practice includes implanting electrical stimulators under the scalp to provide constant low-grade stimulation in an attempt to boost memory function (he also offers patients massage and pedicures), Firlik points out that the ethics behind cognitive enhancement is the one deepening wrinkle. Academics, many of whom have never even spoken to satisfied clients, claim that cognitive enhancement threatens to broaden the socioeconomic gaps in society. Plastic surgery triggered similar debates years ago, but the debates didn't last. (Halpern, 2006, p. 20)

This is one of the perfectly predictable consequences of our pragmatic civilisation. The body always stands in need of greater improvement and the "naturalisation of the mind" always includes on its horizon various techniques for putting an end to ageing and keeping up some hope of immortality. Cosmetic neurosurgery is falling in line with those other bodily techniques that, thanks to science, are prolonging the dreams that Taoist techniques naturalised in ancient China.

The trace of the impossible

In the classic phase of his teaching, Lacan re-read Freud's "Project for a scientific psychology", inspired by the more advanced neurology of his time, considering the Freudian unconscious to be a particular kind of memory: a memory of the impossible. Based on circuits of impossibilities, this memory was compatible with the repetition of traumatic experiences of jouissance and the beyond of the pleasure principle, thus defying homeostasis.[3] Lacan drew his inspiration from the schematisation he had set out in the late 1950s for the functioning of the "reverberating loops" that were being refined by the cyberneticians of the time.

> Lacan [...] took an interest, as we have already seen, in the theory of closed reverberating circuits that Lawrence Kubie's work in the 1930s had led McCulloch to take up, and he was familiar with the work of the British neuro-anatomist John Z. Young [who tested] this theory in the octopus. (Dupuy, 2000, p. 109)[4]

Starting off from these reverberating feedback phenomena, Lacan came to call into question the very possibility of writing the subject's topology into the anatomical support of the living being. It is rather the living being that will come to be caught in a writing of a higher order, in which it finds itself fragmented and parcelled out.

The Freudian unconscious allows for a radical distinction between two levels of experience. First, there is the level of traces of experiences felt by an organism that perceives reality through organs that endue it with an image of this reality: "the living being's insertion into the reality which is what he imagines it to be and which can be gauged by the way it reacts therein" (Lacan, 2001a, p. 334). This register has to be distinguished from the second, which is:

> The subject's bond with a discourse whence he can be suppressed, that is, not knowing that this discourse implies him.
>
> The astounding picture of amnesia that is termed *identity amnesia* ought to be quite edifying here.
>
> [...] The enigma is singled out but that much better given that the subject does not lose any benefit here of what has been learnt. (Lacan, 2001a, p. 334)

In Lacan's late teaching, the unconscious is defined as a form of knowledge that acts directly upon the body of the speaking being. It is a break in the representation of the subject within the signifying system. It is a knowledge of incompatibility between the linguistic system and the body's jouissance, a memory of breaking-points, in some sense. The body emerges from this having been fragmented by a host of different trajectories that are stamped with holes.

> For my part, I say that knowledge affects the body of the being that only becomes Being through words, and does so in fragmenting its jouissance, in thereby slicing it up to the extent of producing off-cuts which I turn into the [...] object *a* [...]. (Lacan, 2001b, p. 550)

The jouissance of the body is not produced by representations of events or by the memory-storage of such events. The memory of the unconscious acts by virtue of the absence of traces. The wanting availability of a signifier signals the irruption of a jouissance that has upset inscription.

> The unconscious is not subliminal, a weak brightness. It is the light which does not make room for shade, nor does contour insinuate itself. It represents my representation right where it is missing, where I am but a lack of the subject. (Lacan, 2001a, p. 334, footnote 1)

Lacan is trusting of what lies outside meaning and is wary of sense, as are our theoreticians of cognition, but this is the reverse of representation conceived of in terms of storage. The locus of the subject is both the locus of loss and the locus of the encounter therewith, the *Tuché*. The unconscious is not the trace of a learning process, it is an interplay with the wanting signifier. "When the space of a lapsus no longer carries any meaning (or interpretation), then only is one sure that one is in the unconscious" (Lacan, 1977b, p. xxxix). This is the foundation of the incommensurable.

What is at stake in the search for inscription is a quest for meaning at a time when so many certainties are falling from under us in the established discourses of our civilisation. As Jacques-Alain Miller has noted, both the body and nature now occupy the place that was erstwhile held by the divine guarantee.

One can also think that all this has its correlate in the mind of God, and that everything we live is recorded there. It is very hard to demonstrate that this is impossible, but this doesn't help at all in practice. (Miller & Etchegoyen, 1996, p. 33)

The main stake in the dialogue with the neurosciences on the incommensurable is to know just how far we can sustain "a theory that embraces a lack that must be met across all levels, inscribing itself hither in indeterminacy, thither in certitude, and forming the nexus of the uninterpretable" (Lacan, 2001a, p. 337). This nexus can also be expressed as follows: what is a discourse that holds together with no other guarantee besides interpretation itself? What is a discourse, like psychoanalysis, which strives to dispense with the semblance of all the guarantees that civilisation offers in response to the troubling question of what it means to speak? The inscription of the subject and of what it is impossible to guarantee in the subject, his naturalisation, are part of this semblance.

Here too they try to reassure us. Once it has been Pavlovised, our anxiety will have no more cause to be. And then we shall be able to hold our silence in a state of appeased animality.

Notes

1. See also, Laroche, S., 2006. The author cites: Castellucci et al., 1970, p. 1745; and Bliss & Lømo, 1973, p. 331.
2. [The published English-language translation of the article is based on a revised text in which the sentence beginning "The homeostatic requirement ..." does not feature. (Tr.)]
3. We would refer the reader to the graph that Lacan includes in the "Seminar on 'The Purloined Letter'" (Lacan, 2006, pp. 35–36).
4. Dupuy is referring to the lesson of 19 January 1955 from *Seminar II*, in which Lacan mentions the octopus in the context of his discussion on memory and the feedback phenomenon (Lacan, 1988, pp. 88–89).

PART II

IMPOSSIBLE EVALUATION

CHAPTER THREE

Collective expert-assessment and compared clinical trials: a machine run amok

B efore reading any of the collective expert-assessment reports issued by the French National Institute for Healthcare and Medical Research (Inserm), it should be noted that the institution enlists all kinds of experts. In those questions bearing on psychoanalysis, it does not seem to have been particularly easy for Inserm to maintain amicable relations with the experts it chose. Consider, for example, the difference between Dr Plantade and Dr Thurin. When Inserm published the document *Troubles mentaux: Dépistage et prévention chez les enfants et l'adolescent* (Inserm, 2002), Plantade was openly critical:

> We know that the sole orientation that was given to this work led three child psychiatrists (who initially formed part of the group of experts) to withdraw, which shows that this work on no account represents a consensus but just one approach to the mental pathology of children. It would have been an honest gesture to inform the reader of this point. (Plantade, 2004)

Dr Plantade belongs to the category of experts who stepped down when the work was in course.

In this respect he took a different path from Dr Thurin, who wittingly opted for a very different policy and chose not to resign from the assessment on *Psychothérapie: trois approches évaluées* (Inserm, 2004, p. 40) so as not to give rise to a text that would be "severed of any psychoanalytic dimension". He confirms, however, that tensions in the group of experts ran very high and animosity towards psychoanalysis was extreme. He is critical of the assessment:

> The results of this assessment call for a rigorous critique, but a move towards evaluation in the fields of the psychoanalytic psychotherapies also needs to be advanced and developed as far as possible. Indeed, some of the bases of such evaluation have already been laid by teams who have not been discouraged in the face of the complexity of this undertaking. My fear is that in the absence of a true awareness of what is currently at stake, psychoanalysis and the psychoanalytic psychotherapies will simply be ejected from the healthcare field [...] Ousting psychoanalysis from the field of Health is without any doubt a dream that a significant number of decision makers currently harbour. (Thurin, 2004a)

Faced with this "evaluate or perish" alternative, Thurin chose, in the chapters he authored, to set out a "toolbox" with which to produce "good" evaluations, evaluations from which psychoanalysis would emerge grander and undiminished. In short, Thurin tells us that he pulled off a Léo Strauss exercise in the art of writing under persecution.

Indeed, we meet many reservations about the assessment project coming from within the assessment team itself. The examples are abundant and they define a veritable rhetoric. For instance, after comparing a number of meta-analyses, the text concludes that the procedure of meta-analysis in itself says nothing, and so it can be made to say many different things: "We can see how meta-analysis can be made to say whatever one wants to hear" (Inserm, 2004, p. 42). On one hand, Thurin affirms:

> The comparative perspective on the effectiveness of psychotherapies that was used in this assessment has now been very widely criticised and abandoned. The authors now recommend an individualised approach rather than an all-encompassing pseudo-response, which moreover was based on methodologies whose limitations and potential bias are well-known. (Thurin, 2004a)

On the other hand, shortly after the assessment was presented to the press, Thurin issued a "postscript" in which he takes a certain distance from this position. He sums up by saying:

> Today it has become possible to evaluate the results of the psycho-analytic psychotherapies on bases that are both scientifically solid and acceptable with respect to the specific objectives of these treat-ments. (Thurin, 2004b)

Thus, he is calling for further assessment. This is a strange pedagogy in which insufficiency coupled with falsehood are supposed to lead to truthfulness.

An insistent pedagogy

Many things have been lumped together under the heading of the said collective expert-assessment report. I shall start by picking out one of the features that typify it: this assessment is a paradoxical pedagogi-cal enterprise. Thurin reads this paradox from his stance of an expert who is at once the relentless propagandist and first critic of the assess-ment. This expert assessment report does not live up to its title. It com-pares utterly distinct approaches in the name of the so-called unity of the psychotherapies. It claims to be speaking about psychoanalytic psychotherapies, when in fact it looks at short-term therapies which have only a vague connection with psychoanalysis and are rarely used in France. Furthermore, it does not compare the therapies with one another in terms of relative effectiveness. It presents some measure-ment of CBT's direct effectiveness on a certain number of "disorders" defined in accordance with the DSM clinical repertoire, and then goes on to present a very small quantity of measurement of the same type carried out by advocates of the "psychodynamic" orientation, who pre-cisely are critical of both the pertinence of the DSM clinic and the per-tinence of measuring direct effectiveness on symptoms that have been simplified, compartmentalised, and cut off from the history of a subject. Underlining this discrepancy between the two currents in their stand-points on measuring, the report concludes with a *woe betide any who will not measure in abiding by our norms, the fault is theirs!* The abundance of statistical explanations by which they present the difference between level-one empirical studies, level-two meta-analyses, and level-three reviews of meta-analyses published in the report, is a smokescreen. It masks over the fact that this is an enterprise designed to do systematic harm to the psychoanalytic orientation. Their examination of the third approach, the "systemic" approach to family therapy, often seems to have been included simply to screen over the full-frontal enterprise of discrediting the psychoanalytic approach; an enterprise which is at work in a variety of disguised forms.

Can one say with Dr Thurin that the assessment "spun out of control" at one point? This would imply admitting that it was fair at the start. It should be noted that the majority of critics who have read this report from the standpoint of the psychodynamic current, albeit on the face of it intimidated by its statistical apparatus, very quickly noticed that the results had been obtained by unacceptable methods. Someone as favourable to quantitative methods as Dr Bernard Brusset, after three months of prudent silence admitted as much (Brusset, 2004). The reasoning that runs: *yes indeed, the method is insufficient, yes indeed, the results are disastrous, but we have to carry on because there will be better studies in the near future,* is hardly very convincing. This is not an appeal to brighter days to come but brighter days to evaluate. They reckon that we will be able to come up with studies that will be capable both of respecting the specificity of our practice and of bringing it in line with quantitative procedures that will demonstrate the effectiveness, even the superiority, of psychodynamic approaches over other approaches. On the whole, it has been hard to convince the psychoanalytic movement of the merits of this. Most practitioners are not particularly thrilled with these perspectives and do not really see any point in participating in this vast evaluative pedagogy in the name of a short-term "measure or perish" ethos.

It is not mere menace that looms large in this pedagogy. It tells us and repeats to us that it is now possible for psychoanalysts to accept quantitative evaluation without any qualms. This used to be difficult, Hans Eysenck having already started, back in 1950, to put in place the evaluative reference with the declared goal of wringing the neck of psychoanalysis. The Inserm assessment team know this full well:

> Levitt's review on evaluating child psychotherapies (1957), which was contemporary with Eysenck's review for adults (1952), came [...] to the same pessimistic conclusion: the traditional forms of psychotherapy are no more effective than an absence of treatment. (Inserm, 2004, p. 43)

At least this declaration had the merit of being frank and direct. In response to this,

> in the 'fifties and 'sixties, the first generation of studies on the effectiveness of psychoanalysis posed the question of their capacity to bring about a modification of the personality, while specifying or differentiating between neither the forms of psychotherapy employed nor the clinical problems to be treated. (Inserm, 2004, pp. 43–44)

This brings us back to our present situation. It is being said that we may take into account the functioning of the person across its different dimensions and, by continually refining the methodology, we may confidently put ourselves in the hands of our friends the evaluators. This is the first of *four modalities*, which I shall now examine, by which confidence in measurement could be generated. We are being exhorted to measure because it is possible, so they assert, beyond the short-sighted measurement of effectiveness on compartmentalised, divided-up symptoms that have been removed from their subjective context: to measure therapeutic effectiveness on the functioning of the person as a whole in the context of an effective and complex practice; to produce measurement that shows that what is at issue is indeed the psychodynamic process; and to see psychotherapy finally taking up its legitimate place among the other therapies.

Symptom and function

The first modality is the affirmation which holds that it is now possible not only to measure *effectiveness on the symptom* by means of questionnaires and the ubiquitous tick-box, but also the *functioning of the person* across a whole variety of "functions". This was an ideal that was first put in place by Robert Knight (Knight, 1941) after the Marienbad Congress and which was taken up again in the 1990s. This position underwrote a whole stream of thought in the Société psychanalytique de Paris, which sought, via object relations, to define a sort of characterology of the subject, of his characterological armour, which could be objectified and measured. We have a trace of this in published form in the 1955 volume *La psychanalyse d'aujourd'hui*. Lacan opposed this stream in maintaining on the contrary that one should not move in the direction of greater objectification but rather, as he argues in his study on "The direction of the treatment and the principles of its power", towards greater subjectification (Lacan, 2006, pp. 489–542).

The path towards the objectification of the person's functioning was pursued both inside and outside France. So it was that in 1995 we met a reformulation of these objectives which was barely modified with respect to what had been announced in 1941:

> [...] different studies have associated with comprehensive dimensions (demographic and sanitary variables) the evaluation of symptoms (research into a specific or systematic pathology), the evaluation of personal functioning (in particular with respect to social relations and *passages à l'acte*), and the measurement of dimensions of acquisition such as construction of the self, maturation, consciousness and awareness of conflicts in reality, quality of object relations, affective capacities, ability to carry out work, or access to affects and their integration in the personality (Monson et al., 1955). (Inserm, 2004, p. 78)

In this report, Dr Thurin further announces that, despite the dearth of evaluative studies in French, our colleagues from the thirteenth arrondissement of Paris are preparing a soon-to-be-published study:

> It is worthwhile pointing out the work of a group of French psychiatrists [...] from the Mental Health Association in Arrondissement 13 [...] which has devised a scale for the evaluation of chronic psychotic states based on a psychoanalytic comprehension of mental pathology. This scale draws on a study of the entirety of the patient's situation: detailed clinical state, social situation, impact of disorders on the family, relationship with the care system, and physical state. It uses semiological groupings of conduct, ascertainment of mental functioning, and written impressions from the care teams in their observation of the patient himself and his interactions with his family and social surroundings. (Inserm, 2004, pp. 79–80)

That's rather a lot. And one can't help thinking that these questionnaires must be fairly hefty. In one institution, educators recently had to answer a questionnaire numbering 900 items listed on a stack of pages that constituted a small volume. One can always go down this path of refining further and further, going off to fill out not 200 but 300 pages no sooner than the patient arrives. Indeed, from this perspective they are delighted at the fact that "based on the scoring of 85 patients by an average of four raters, inter-rater reliability was evaluated and deemed to be satisfying for this scale" (Inserm, 2004, p. 80).

The limitation of this approach is quite simple. From the point of view of the evaluators, it will never be adequate. There will always need to be more pages, more time spent filling in questionnaires and ticking boxes. And to obtain what?

The evaluators will always be able at some point to make concessions to the psychodynamic practitioners, just as was done for the DSM. They will consent to an axis II, in which one will be able to include the patient's functioning, so that should anyone object to an objectification that is rather troubling, we will be told that the axis II will take care of everything, including the objections. We shall just have to fill out another thirty-odd pages. I daresay this is not a particularly fruitful path.

Context: simplification and complexity

The second modality of legitimisation concerns the difficulty in accounting for the context of clinical effectiveness, which now purportedly lies within the scope of the quantitative studies. Where do we start if we are to move towards a means of accounting for context? Let's look at one study mentioned in the assessment that reports on the results of short-term psychotherapy (Strupp & Hadley, 1979):

> A relatively homogenous population of 49 students between 17 and 24 years of age who were either depressed or psychasthenic according to the MMPI [Minnesota Multiphasic Personality Inventory], and who had been recruited through a poster campaign and via consultants in the healthcare service, were entrusted in part to professional psychotherapists of psychoanalytic orientation and in another part to teachers selected on the basis of their reputation for empathy and the trust they inspired in the students. The "control" group was made up of students on the waiting list. The therapy was limited to 25 hours over a period of 3 to 4 months, at a rate of two sessions per week. The results show that the patients who had psychotherapy with the teachers presented, on average,

improvement that is as significantly important as the patients treated by experienced professional therapists. (Inserm, 2004, p. 80)

What is going on here? This recruitment of students on university campuses by means of posters is not a therapeutic matter but some kind of academic game, a parody of university life that would not be out of place on the pages of David Lodge's *Paradise News*, in its comic aspect. Its more tragic aspect is more reminiscent of J. M. Coetzee. This is a cruel game that boils down to manipulating transference in an academic setting.

Likewise, the cases of our CBT colleagues remain strangely unreal when mention is made of them. They are mere shadows standing in for a category, whilst their presence such as they appear in the accounts remains extremely ghostly. Their most enlightened advocates state their case rather awkwardly. For example, in the newspaper *Le Monde*, professor Quentin Debray advocates the possibility of behavioural treatment for chronic fatigue by selectively limiting the tasks to be carried out, accompanied by highly active suggestion. At the same time, he pre-empts his defence by saying:

> Some psychoanalyst colleagues judge these therapies to be some-what simplistic. First of all, this is not altogether true, because their application can be subtle and nuanced.

This sentence is crucial. It shows that Debray is the advocate of one particular type of CBT. Indeed, there is a conflict between those who think that the therapy handbooks should be adapted to the case, and those who insist that people with the least possible qualification should follow the handbooks to the letter. In the latter case, the less qualified they are, the more likely they are to follow the procedure word for word. These two approaches are very distinct. Two options set them apart. Those who advocate *adaptation* insist on the necessity of training. They are the supporters of a prerequisite of training in psychopathology which they would like to control. On the other hand, those who accentuate *automaticity* are undoubtedly the same who want to appropriate these therapies so as then to delegate them, under strict control, to low-qualified personnel.

The "virtual" aspect of measurement that is supposed to approximate a way of accounting for the context and the effectiveness of clinical activity is constantly showing itself in new colours. The wide gap between the abundant presentations of statistics from meta-analyses and the effective content of what is being measured is often quite staggering. For example, with respect to the meta-analysis by Smith and Glass who back in 1980 collected for the first time some 475 studies on 25,000 subjects, one of the many criticisms that was levelled at them was that pooling together these different studies effectively placed on the same level work that was undertaken with volunteering students and work undertaken with real patients. This is one of the reasons that the conclusions did not reflect the reality of modern-day clinical practice. In actual fact, 22% of them were real patients, the other 78% were students recruited using attractive posters. In the end, in the expert report, when they want to measure effectiveness on symptoms, they note that the only method that has a significant effect (i.e., higher than 0.80) is "systematic desensitisation". They present no questioning of this tautology, which effectively affirms that to make a symptom disappear the most direct method is to disgust the subject with his symptom. It consists of more or less cruel ways of either exposing him to the traumatic or phobic object, or forbidding his rituals, which are subjected to strong coercion. Even the die-hard advocates of measurement acknowledge the limitations of this approach in a context that has not been artificialised by the methods we have just looked at.

Peter Fonagy in the UK, who has become a specialist in "context" measurement, has a psychoanalytic training and has been searching with precision for the right methodology. He observes that for schizophrenias treated in hospital the treatments are so multi-factorial that it is hard to measure just one element. How can one neglect the fact that there exist multi-therapies and that interventions cannot be limited to just one psychotherapy? There is the pharmacotherapy, there are the effects of the institution, and so on and so forth. All this means that measuring effectiveness poses enormous problems when it comes to execution, analysis, presentation and interpretation. The meta-analyses merely amplify the problem. Fonagy does manage to give some results for "borderline" patients because the institutions that care for them are much lighter in structure and the follow-up can be done outside the institution. One can therefore say that in the case of borderline patients it is possible to adapt the treatment to the measurement. In fact, the only thing that one really measures is not so much the effectiveness of the treatment on these patients as the fact that the treatment lends itself to the systems of measure.

Symptom and process

Let's look now at the third justification: the argument for measuring the process beyond the result. This argument asserts that it would be possible for psychoanalysis to consent to this kind of measurement because it would be possible to measure effective process in the resolution of the symptom. With this, psychoanalytic method could be measured. From this perspective, Lester Luborsky in the 1980s developed a handbook of principles of analytic psychotherapy for "expression" and "support" treatments. It is drafted in such a way that the hypotheses that it implements can be measured with the aid of a few simple variables. The term "process" is ostensibly being used to validate the psychoanalytic concepts (such as the unconscious, fantasy, transference, and interpretation) in their very application. He believed it would thereby exorcise the objection that is levelled at all "handbook-free" psychotherapy, namely, the "Dodo Bird Verdict".

The Dodo Bird Verdict debate came to the fore some thirty years ago, in the wake of the results of a meta-analysis by Gene Glass, the inventor of the term "meta-analysis" (Cialdella, 2007). The label Dodo Bird Verdict is in homage to Lewis Carroll. In *Alice's Adventures in Wonderland*, a number of animal characters become dripping wet and want to get dry again. They begin by telling "dry" stories, but this doesn't work. Then the dodo suggests a Caucus-Race, but no one knows what that is.

> [...] when they had been running half an hour or so, and were quite dry again, the Dodo suddenly called out "The race is over!" and they all crowded round it, panting, and asking, "But who has won?" [...] "*EVERYBODY* has won, and all must have prizes." (Carroll, 1865, Ch. III)

In the measurement of psychotherapies that focus on symptoms, some claim that the theory that underwrites these therapies is never measured. All of them are equally good because none of them are accurate. Therefore, there is no point in measuring with any precision the action of whichever psychotherapy is in question.[1]

In reaction to this came the idea of developing a straightforward handbook for expression and support therapies. In passing from fundamental concepts to measurable items, however, the essence of the concepts is lost; but still, the Department of Counselling in the American Psychological Association is in the process of studying a mode of quantitative evaluation for therapies that do not seek to reduce things to a specific diagnostics. They contrast their "process"-based interventions with the outcome-focused CBT methods.

> Therapies such as psychodynamic, experiential, and existential are "process oriented," whereas CBT is more "outcome oriented". That is, in CBT, the goal is to modify the psychiatric disorder or its symptoms as directly and efficiently as possible. The process-oriented therapies, on the other hand, view symptomatic changes as occurring indirectly through exploration of emergent themes, schemas, or unconscious motives and beliefs. (Messer, 2002)

Therefore, they address the "therapist-client relationship qualities and therapist stances that enhance therapy progress and outcome". The essential thing is that they should manage to present their results in terms of "empirically supported relationships".

So as to measure the "process", they include the transference in the operation:

> Practice and treatment guidelines should explicitly address therapist behaviours and qualities that promote a facilitative therapy relationship; [...] the therapeutic relationship acts in concert with [...] patient characteristics and clinician qualities in determining the treatment effectiveness. A comprehensive understanding of effective (and ineffective) psychotherapy will consider all of these determinants and their optimal combinations; and adapting or tailoring the therapy relationship to the specific patient needs and characteristics (in addition to diagnosis) enhances the effectiveness of the treatment. (Messer, 2002)

Who can believe in this version of transference reduced to a kind of virtuality, a sort of potentiating virtue of effectiveness?

Downscaling psychotherapy to the level of a drug

Within this perspective they deem it crucial, not to bring out the particularity of the "psychotherapy" object, but to reduce it to the paradigm that governs all therapy: medication. In the conclusion to the first section of the report, the authors show us perfectly the steps through which this object is reformulated:

> In conclusion, the age of carrying out broad comparisons of psychotherapeutic methods, applied to various psychopathological disturbances, which are pooled together and which entail voluntary participation, is now over. The current strategy is, for each disorder defined by the ICD or the DSM, to take certain types of psychotherapy that have been well-defined in an operational manner and to compare them with a placebo and with medical treatments. (Inserm, 2004, p. 44)

The fact of introducing this comparison with medication alone is a crucial step. It could be considered to be an incongruity: how would it be pertinent to include medication in the evaluation of a psychotherapy? This point is crucial because it actually allows for a justification of a new method: the compared clinical trial. One of the experts, a supporter of CBT, underlines the novelty of this:

> This is the beginning of studies that allocate subjects at random to one of the different treatments under comparison. Since the 1980s, the third generation of research in psychotherapy has been using the model of controlled clinical trials imported from pharmacotherapy, along with DSM diagnostics and handbooks describing precisely which treatments to use. (Inserm, 2004, pp. 43–44)

For the clinical trials used in pharmacopoeia, however, homogeneous populations are required, along with randomisation and a control group that is issued a placebo or "reference treatment" (Pignarre, 2001, pp. 56–57). These two criteria are not respected in the studies we are looking at here. How is one to ensure straightforwardness in diagnostics? "The main stumbling block of meta-analytic studies is the pooling together of studies on various different pathologies or psychological problems" (Inserm, 2004, p. 41). Furthermore, seek as they might to break any possible transference by means of authoritarian randomisation, this is one effect that seems to be impossible to eliminate as soon as you set up a subject-supposed-to-know. The study cited above, contrasting "nice teachers" with "competent to professionals", shows this very well. Moreover, in his report Thurin lets it be known that

> two criteria for excellence currently seem to be inapplicable to
> research on dynamic psychotherapies: the direct application of the
> treatment handbooks and authoritarian randomisation of patients
> into different treatment groups. (Inserm, 2004, p. 97)

These "criteria for excellence" are merely criteria for inclusion in the
compared clinical-trial procedure. This inclusion is a key step in reporting on psychotherapies within the wide catch-all category of evaluation
by means of the compared clinical-trial method.

Having initially been invented to curb the power of the pharmaceutical industry, this method has become the chief motor behind the pressure that laboratories now routinely apply so as to obtain by any means
necessary the authorisation to put their products on the market. By all
accounts this is a machine that is now running at full tilt.

> Nothing seems to be able to limit the model's inventiveness, even
> though it stands independent of any creation of reliable witnesses.
> The psychiatric biology that accompanies this process is essen-
> tially a biology of bio-chemical receptors in the brain: it provides
> explanations on how psychotropics act, it helps in selecting new
> psychotropics from among the drugs that are available in the
> pharmaceutical industry's chemical library, but it cannot claim to
> provide a causal explanation for mental disturbances. It does not
> merit the name "biology". We would recommend calling this set
> of techniques *minor biology*. [...] This procedure pushes to its tri-
> umphant conclusion the fact that a modern drug is invariably the
> next-to-latest one. There will always be another drug that is more
> effective, more manageable, and less toxic. This "minor biology"
> gladly decks itself out in the trimmings of biology *per se*, but its
> ambitions are limited to the development of new drugs that will
> always be next-to-latest. (Pignarre, 2001, pp. 81–82)

We have a recent example of the demented functioning of this system
in the effectiveness assessments of the panacea Omega-3. An article by
Paul Benkimoun reports on this:

> Have the Omega-3 fatty acids proven to be scientifically effective?
> [...] There exists great enthusiasm and a "hype" effect, but the
> scientific basis for Omega-3's action on depression is still rather

weak: six studies including a total of 200 people. With just one
exception, these studies associated Omega-3 with a treatment by
antidepressants for the full duration of the trial, even if it was
not proving to be effective. [...] Furthermore, the published studies do not provide any information on the mid-term effects of the
Omega-3 supplement, let alone its effects in the long term. Do the
beneficial effects last? Do harmful effects set in? At present it is not
possible to assert that taking Omega-3 polyunsaturated fatty acids
is capable of preventing the emergence of depressive disturbances
or of avoiding their relapse. To be able to do so, it is indispensable
to provide studies carried out with a serious methodology, with a
significant sufferer population, and over sufficiently long duration.
(Benkimoun, 2004, p. 26)

The mountain of studies has thus brought forth a mouse: *let's do more
research*. Here we have a perfect description of "research" formatted by
these methods and by the rhetoric of evaluation. Why then give oneself over to a game that has been lost before it even begins? It can only
be that what is being measured in these studies is something else: the
transformation of the object of psychoanalysis once it has been taken up
in the problematic of evaluation.

Comparing the incomparable, ceaselessly creating new equivalence
ratings in the name of the homogenisation of measurement, permits of
reducing the phenomenological remainder known as "the personality"
to a mere cluster of comorbidity. In this sense, "comorbidity" is precisely the concept that permits of reducing a subject's entire pathology
to a mere disorder with no opportunity for protest. The supporters of
CBT insist that one symptom cannot come in the stead of another once
the target symptom has been treated. If a new symptom should emerge
it is due to the comorbidity of several disorders that are finding successive expression. If we add to this the category of "residual disturbances"
which has gained acceptance in CBT studies, we find that the complexity of the symptom and its plasticity has been translated into a language
that allows it to be upheld as something that cannot be substituted.

To evaluate the long-term effectiveness of CBT in obsessive-
compulsive disorders, the results of 9 studies of (controlled) group
studies were colligated. From a follow-up of 1 to 6 years (3 years
on average), a 78% improvement rate was shown with an average

> reduction in rituals of 60%. However, residual symptoms were
> the rule and the risk of depression was unchanged. (Inserm, 2004,
> p. 503)

And yet the defenders of CBT assert that within their paradigm the symptom remains one sole entity that cannot be replaced. They assert this quite adamantly because it is one of the cornerstones of their system. The symptom cannot be replaced, but the therapists (who have been rapidly trained and who are, in practice, no one in particular) can (so long as they are closely controlled and monitored). The collective-expert assessment we are examining here seeks to share with us, in the name of CBT, the reductionist passion that drives these experts.

They also need to explain how, on the basis of these simplified disorders and reductive treatments, one is able to observe repercussions across the subject's life as a whole. The non-measurable effect created by this treatment is called its "ripple effect", an effect that reaches out like wavelets on the surface of water. It evaluates any effect caused by a therapy focused on one symptom that extends beyond this one symptom: "behavioural therapy has effects that are both specific and deeper and dispersed" and "this phenomenon is comparable to the propagation of a wave" (Inserm, 2004, p. 38). This effectiveness, which extends beyond the limits, which reaches beyond the bounds of the specific disturbance, is a source of great delight to CBT therapists. It does indicate a problem, however, which is reminiscent of the problem of ether in pre-Einstein physics. What medium is supposed to support the wave that is transmitted? By definition, this can only be the consciousness of the patient. So, what is that? Is it a form of cognitive-behavioural unconscious? An immobile and homogeneous ether with no other property besides that of accommodating this ripple effect produced by the treatment of the symptom?

In these reductionist procedures, which have been scaled-down in the name of measurement, what remains of the fantasy as an indicator of relationships with the Other? It is taken into account in scales that measure "interpersonal problems and their relation to styles of attachment". Next, they evaluate

> problems of amiable submissiveness ("I find it hard to say 'no' to
> someone") that seem to be more difficult to treat with short-term
> dynamic psychotherapy than problems of hostile dominance

("I find it hard to commit to someone on a long-term basis" or "I find it hard to put my trust in another person"). [...] The results also suggest relationships between a person's type of interpersonal problem and his or her principal attachment style (secure, preoccupied, fearful, deserting). (Inserm, 2004, p. 85)

In the same spirit, Jean-François Allilaire has noted that in the US no one speaks about transference anymore, but rather inter-subjective relations.[2]

Once everything has been subjected to this kind of Jivaroan head-shrinking rite, what else is there left to do but modify the patient in accordance with the measurement? This is exactly what a team of researchers in California have set out to perform:

Vaughan et al. carried out a feasibility study designed to research into whether patients in psychodynamic treatment, including psychoanalysis, could be recruited and maintained as subjects for studies; to determine patient and therapist compliance to take part in evaluative measuring by means of questionnaires, structured interviews and recorded sessions; and to obtain pilot data on changes in these measurements after one year of treatment. (Inserm, 2004, p. 93)

Evidently, this feasibility study only succeeded in enrolling a very small number of people (nine patients in psychoanalysis and fifteen patients in twice-weekly psychodynamic psychotherapy).

In Germany, at the initiative of the German Society of the International Psycho-analytic Association (DPV), they went about things in the opposite way, retrospectively rather than prospectively, evaluating

the patients' retrospective views of their experiences with psychoanalytic therapy and its effects more than four years after the end of their psychoanalyses or long-term psychoanalytic therapies. [...] Two sorts of data were examined: i. Extra-analytic data bearing on symptoms, changes in capacity to cope with life events, self-esteem, mood, and life satisfaction, alongside a general evaluation of their therapy, their work ability, and any recourse to healthcare services; ii. Analytic data assessing in particular the transference and countertransference reactions, and free association, leading to analyses of content. (Inserm, 2004, p. 92)

The Germans reacted with great discipline:

> This research entailed first securing the agreement of the psycho-analysts, who declared themselves to be 89% in favour of the study. The second step was to determine a representative sample of all the patients in long-term psychoanalytic treatment during this period, and this did not present any recruitment problems either ($n = 401$). (Inserm, 2004, p. 92)

What they were asking for, however, was somewhat complex: recorded interviews and detailed or semi-detailed questionnaires. The interviews (two for each former patient plus a third with the former analyst) were recorded and discussed by a research group.

There was no discussion whatsoever about the constitution of the lists, about the suspension of confidentiality, about the former patients' eagerness to respond, about the setting-up of this panopticon, nor about the perverse practice of getting people to speak about their analysis in this rash and foolhardy imitation of the procedure of the Pass. This high cost was paid only to yield the following paltry results:

> The most remarkable evolution was that 84.3% of the former patients were climbing the social ladder. Furthermore, they had internalised their analytic attitude, thereby rendering themselves capable of pursuing the analytic process after the end of their treatment.

The rest is of much the same calibre.

Researchers in German-speaking Switzerland are preparing to carry out a study of the same ilk with the blessing of the current IPA authorities. In France, a recent text has called for studies based on effective practice and testimony from former patients: "It is a matter of objectifying what corresponds to present-day clinical experience and to numerous testimonies from former patients of psychoanalysts" (Brusset, 2004).

The way that Europe is following on from the United States in this kind of evaluative study carries its own particularity. It is tacking on assessment-manager bureaucracy (Miller & Milner, 2004). Never in the US have they enrolled patients who have done an analysis in chores such as the Germans have set or certain French researchers are seeking to set.

The dead end of short-term measurement policy

What then is driving the European psychoanalytic movement onto the path of making ever more concessions to the measurers in the hope of obtaining a share of the psychotherapy market by means of the academic machinery of CBT?

The new balance in the supply of care in France being proposed by some of the experts who drafted the Inserm report amounts to the administrative constitution of a new order in the supply of psychotherapy (Swendsen, 2004). The supply being sought by the representatives of cognitive-behavioural therapy in state institutions is an odd blend, heavy on the CBT and light on the psychoanalysis. The press releases from associations of CBT practitioners in the wake of the publication of the Inserm report have been moving in this direction.

We are not the only ones to voice concern over these leanings towards an administrative modification of the supply of care. Brusset too is worried about the consequences of CBT homogenisation:

> Cognitive-behavioural therapies, which are low-cost because they are short and can be carried out by paramedical staff, have in their favour the fact of their rapid effectiveness in suppressing symptoms, but the indications for them are limited and cannot be extended without the risk of later complications. (Brusset, 2004)

He notes that, therefore, "there is cause for concern in various reports initiated by the government over the direct or indirect promotion of these techniques for the short-term suppression of symptoms" and draws our attention to the long-term cost. Dr Christian Vasseur has threatened Inserm that he will turn to France's national advisory council on bioethics issues (CCNE) should the report be published:

> This study, which has already been printed in the popular press, should be reconsidered prior to any use whatsoever since it poses methodological problems for both scientificity and the deepening of ethical reflection. Should this not be the case and an impatient decision-maker should make use of it, we shall interpellate the

CCNE with the support of a responsible political representative as was recently and usefully the case for the issue of "psychosurgery". Ethical and moral reflection is called upon by psychotherapeutic action when the threat of reductionism looms as large as it does here. (Vasseur, 2004)

Beyond these reactions on these precise points, it would seem that a wider point of inflection is perceptible in the reactions to the short-term scientistic arguments. There is great convergence in the oppositions that are being levelled from all quarters at this system for having obeyed the imperatives of the new "biological" approach in psychiatry. The new stranglehold of the ideology of measurement, the new push in what Dominique Laurent has called a "desire for mass standardisation" (Laurent, 2004), is coming up against a movement of disenchantment and resistance.

The psychiatric clinic of the DSM should be viewed as neither evidence nor proof. Twenty years after its first application, its effects are being criticised, as is the slide towards evidence-based medicine that we have seen across the medical field as a whole. During the European Congress on Classification and Diagnosis organised by the World Health Organization and the World Association of Psychiatry in London on 12–13 July 2001, diverging positions were voiced, precisely on the nature and use of the current classifications. The goals set by the promoters of the DSM clinic have shown themselves to be unattainable. They have only succeeded in making the diagnoses uniform. They have not managed to have them validated by the community of clinicians at large.

The classifications adopted by the WHO and the American Psychiatric Association (APA) have not succeeded in meeting the objectives for which they were created. Between the WHO codifications [the ICD-10 scale] and those of the APA, there are notable differences. Across many regions of the world, both are being shunned in favour of local codifications. Clinicians and researchers in countries that officially abide by one or the other of these classifications dispute, refuse, or bypass many of the items that have been sanctioned. DSM-IV prefers the label "Mood Disorders" for what in DSM-III-R were called "Affective Disorders", and in the ICD-10, "Mood (Affective) Disorder". Goodwin prefers to speak of "manic-depressive illness". Others maintain that these are not clinical categories and that it would be correct to speak of an "affective-disorder spectrum". [...] The entity "dysthymia" is held by some to be a misunderstood concept: a name given to neurotic depression, depressive personalities, and neurasthenia. For others it forms part of the affective illnesses or else represents one dimension of the personality and a sub-affective disorder (Akiskal, 1994). (Sonenreich, 2004a)

The same questions about shoehorning different notions into *categories, entities, disorders* and *spectra* are being posed for all the classifications since psychiatry does not have at its disposal any "reliable biological witness" for each of these entities.

A recent article published in the *American Journal of Psychiatry* takes up these criticisms and constitutes for us a sort of summary of the previous work that calls these codifications into question. Kendell and Jablensky note the disenchantment of the various authors with respect to the revolutionary nosology put forward by the DSM-III and its successors. In fact this nosology has not given rise to any etiological knowledge on any syndrome whatsoever. These codifications are based on aberrant principles (the idea of being "atheoretical"). They justify their eagerness to unify diagnostics by the hope they place in a reliability which has never been reached, in spite of the democratic progress in this direction. They have been seeking to validate the syndromes by means of experimental research. This has not come to fruition. Thus the concept of "validity", as confusingly defined as it is, has had to be abandoned in favour of "utility". [...] They have not managed to avoid the falsification of results that surreptitiously conform to the authors' political or economic interests without demonstrating anything that could be considered to be scientifically meaningful. (Sonenreich, 2004a)[3]

These last criticisms do not mean that the authors wish for a return to the "psychopathology" of old, which indeed they reject wholesale as being scientifically unfounded. They believe that we should now be moving forward to another level, one that is truly scientific. They think we should be searching for correlations along supplementary lines of research: molecular genetics, molecular biology, neurochemistry, neuroanatomy, neurophysiology and cognitive neuroscience.

The contradictions expressed at the London Congress have pushed back the publication date for the next edition of the DSM (which is usually revised every seven years) because of the need for "empirical validations". No new edition will be published before 2012.[4] But make no mistake: we can now say that the political goal of the DSM research programme has been reached. It has made a clean sweep of the clinical field by destroying classical psychopathology. The "scientists" claim that they no longer require psychopathology. It is not so sure, however, that they really require a true biological foundation for their system. Dr Carol Sonenreich observes quite rightly how the multiple research activities seem to feed themselves, without producing much in the way of results besides adding their activities to others while consistently failing to meet their objectives. In actual fact, as Pignarre notes, they contribute towards making people forget that all psychiatry can perfectly well make do without any effective biological validation.

A misunderstanding now unites the advocates of a true biological psychiatry and the supporters of a psychopathology founded on psychoanalysis. For both camps, the DSM clinic no longer enjoys necessity or prestige.

To obtain "inter-rater reliability", which is merely concordance between classifications, the relation to the real has been sacrificed. In attempting to salvage the classifications, their effective relation to anything whatsoever has been increasingly sacrificed. On this point, we follow Sonenreich's critique of DSM diagnostics:

> We do not conduct diagnoses by tallying up symptoms and ignoring their signification. We do not deem empirical research to be an absolute and infallible scientific guarantee above any suspicion. We do not hold the unification of diagnostics to be more important than their validation. A good many nosological entities sanctioned by the ICD and the DSM do not strike us as having been carefully thought through and are of service to neither clinical practice nor clinical research. (Sonenreich, 2004b)

Evidence-based medicine, which has dominated since the 1990s, is itself starting to show its limits. It sought to modify radically the hierarchy of proof in medicine: instead of proceeding on a case-by-case basis as in traditional clinical method, the hierarchy was to be based on statistical studies and meta-analyses. The movement had its origins in Canada, but the Scots became its chief propagators in the United Kingdom (Sackett et al., 1997). Its charter may be defined thus:

> The new hierarchy of evidence places the meta-analysis of random trials at the top; in second place comes the compared randomised study; in third place the controlled study without randomisation; fourthly, a study that is at least partially experimental; fifthly, non-experimental descriptive studies; and in sixth place, expert accounts and opinions of authority. According to this new hierarchy of evidence, the account of an individual case may only be published in an academic journal worthy of the name in its "Letters" section. (Sonenreich, 2004b)

A study published in 2002 by Brazil's Federal Medical Council has questioned this approach. It looks at articles published in journals from the US, Europe, Canada and Australia. One of the examples it criticises concerns olanzapine, the atypical antipsychotic. A review of the meta-analyses proves at the same time that the medication does not cause tardive dyskinesia, that in some patients it can improve dyskinesia caused by other drugs, and that it does cause tardive dyskinesia. These contradictions have, therefore, led to particular cases being taken into account: clinically observed cases that present dyskinesia under the influence of olanzapine.

> The medication approved by EBM was later deemed inappropriate. The value of Lithium, which has been perfectly proven medically and for many is the gold standard for research, has been declared utterly ineffective by studies that conform to EBM. [...] EBM is being used to intimidate, to refuse trade appellations, to apply material sanctions, and so on. Care based on cost/profit calculation will never succeed in defining a better psychiatry. Statistical data, closely linked as they are with EBM, are problematic with potential errors in the definition of categories and the matching of evidence. In practice, the conclusions are incorporated into the scale of facts. (Sonenreich, 2004a)

The recent debates on rofecoxib[5] and celecoxib[6] and this new class of anti-inflammatory drugs, along with the debates on antidepressants, make these contradictions even more acute. Faced with the bias introduced by the meta-analyses and the withdrawal of clinical judgement that it entails, the last message from the out-going president of the American Psychiatric Association, Daniel Borenstein, was an appeal not to let the notion of EBM "proof" sweep aside clinical judgement (Borenstein, 2001, p. 3). This kind of reaction has led psychiatrists to restore qualitative approaches to their former honour and to publish a *Handbook of Qualitative Research* (Denzin & Lincoln, 2000).

So it is that we are seeing a movement taking shape that refuses the novel imperatives of the new approach, whether in medicine, in psychiatry, or in universities and institutions. This movement is in line with the movement that got underway in psychoanalysis following Jacques-Alain Miller's determined refusal of the Accoyer Amendment on 25 October 2003 (Miller, 2005).[7] It defines a policy of refusal to adapt to the world of all-pervasive measurement. In this way, we will be helping the adepts of these new norms of measurement to recognise the limitations of their approach and to scale down their pernicious certainties.

Truth-pulling machinery

The cognitive-behavioural therapies have submitted wholesale to the dictates of measurement and consider that they should be rewarded for and justified by the excellent results they are being accorded by certain studies, for which the Inserm expert report has served as a sounding board. In actual fact, they have merely submitted to the hazards of measure and the inevitable "next study". As I bring this article to a close, a textbook case has just demonstrated this in devastating fashion. On 3 June 2004, we saw the publication of the results of the first study carried out by the USA's National Institute for Mental Health comparing the treatment of depressed teenagers with psychotherapy or Prozac. These results were especially eagerly anticipated because they were produced by an independent national agency and not by a laboratory. This investigation, titled "Treatment for Adolescents with Depression Study", included 439 adolescents from the ages of twelve to seventeen suffering from moderate to severe depression (Harris, 2004). They were given, at random, Prozac, a CBT treatment, placebo pills, or a combination of Prozac and CBT, for a thirty-six week (nine-month) period. According to one scale, the results show that after twelve weeks 71% of subjects receiving the combination of Prozac and CBT were responding well to the treatment, 61% to Prozac alone, 43% to CBT alone, and 35%

to the placebo. According to another rating scale, the placebo and CBT were strictly equivalent.

Regardless of the disparity in the results, the fact of receiving treatment, the fact of not leaving subjects to their own devices, whatever the treatment may be, made these subjects less suicidal. The risk of a suicide attempt was, however, twice as high among those who were prescribed Prozac as among those who did not receive it. These troubling results are in line with recent studies published in the UK, which show that the disinhibitory effect produced by antidepressants at the start of treatment, or else the effects produced when coming off the drug, can lead to a *passage à l'acte* in some subjects. This study, carried out by the UK Department of Health, concluded that the GlaxoSmithKline laboratories (the British manufacturer of the antidepressant paroxetine)[8] had suppressed four studies that highlight the risks of prescribing antidepressants to children. Leaning on this same study, Eliot Spitzer, then Governor of New York State, accused the laboratory of defrauding consumers (Gilpin, 2004). The British health minister took two measures: on one hand banning the prescription of any drug save Prozac as an antidepressant for children, on the other hand, recommending frequent appointments with the doctor during the first weeks of prescription and during the withdrawal phase.

It is in this context that the American study reassures the doctors, who were fearing malpractice suits: the effectiveness of prescription has been proven in "good practice". Millions of cases are potentially implicated in this. On the other hand, the study lays waste to the hopes raised by the results of expert reports such as the Inserm collective. This time, the experts are concluding that CBT, presented as a psychotherapy and a "talk therapy", is no more effective than the placebo. CBT and "psychotherapy" alike find themselves effectively discredited as a treatment in this study.

On 8 June, an article in *The New York Times* afforded an insight into the unease that is being felt across the field (Carey, 2004). How is one to go about reassuring both the parents and the patient, and to help them to choose faced with the risks presented by antidepressants and with the ineffectiveness of the psychotherapies represented by CBT? The special reporter seeks to reassure parents of depressed teenagers by observing that the results are less discouraging than they seem. After all, psychotherapy by CBT did have an effect on 43% of the patients, which is slightly higher than the 35% effect of the placebo. Furthermore, a number of professors of psychiatry in the US have stood up to defend CBT, underlining how large-scale investigations do not account for individual differences. Some insist on particular cases, arguing that results actually depend much more on the case and the therapist than on comprehensive statistics. Some of the best results are not, therefore, taken into account. Others accentuate the preventative benefits of psychotherapies. Others still remind us that a study carried out on 378 cases shows the effectiveness of Prozac to the point of now dispensing with any counselling prior to prescription. And then yet others maintain that in cases of depression in reaction to an affective loss, better to opt for an "interpersonal therapy" which is effective with teenagers. Some suspect that teenagers are too susceptible to their emotions to have the auto-observational attitude that it takes for CBT. They submit less to the note-taking duties and the continuous self-monitoring. So as to come to a close and provide some peace of mind, the article concludes that one should both prescribe and speak on a regular basis, especially given the suicide risk.

It is in this context that we also have to set the disparity in rules for the prescription of antidepressants, given that the good-practice guidelines are supposed to resolve any contradiction. The reader might care to refer to Anne Castot's July 2004 interview with Guy Hugnet.[9] At the present time the prescription guidelines vary from country to country, with discrepancies that are often poorly justified. In the UK, they have just banned the use of paroxetine for under-eighteens,

> while in the US they have settled for a warning, without prohibiting its use. In France, this drug is contraindicated for under-fifteens, but authorised in older teenagers and adults. (Hugnet, 2004, p. 51)

The French Agency for the Safety of Health Products acknowledges the fact and replies:

> In France, Paroxetine has always been contraindicated for under-fifteens. Upwards of sixteen years of age, the reference is the results on adults. At the European level, there is an imbalance. This is why the Brussels Commission should soon be bringing legislation into line across the European member states. […] It will be recommended to avoid using Paroxetine for under-eighteens, but without an absolute ban. The choice should be left to the prescribing doctor.

> Depending on the benefit/risk assessment for any given patient,
> the doctor will be able to prescribe as a last resort if there is no other
> solution. (Hugnet, 2004, p. 201)

At the time of writing, Benedict Carey in *The New York Times* has just presented a summary of the current debate on the safety of antidepressants, which is now shifting to use in adults (Carey, 2005). A study by the University of Ottawa finds that the risk of suicide attempts is double in patients taking antidepressants, although the risk of death by suicide is no higher. Two further studies from the UK find on the contrary that there is no significant risk of increase in suicide. All three studies were posted on the online edition of the *British Medical Journal* on 18 February 2005, in advance of publication in the print edition (Cipriani et al., 2005, pp. 373–374). The journal appeals to the clinical judgement of practitioners and to the utilitarian good sense of patients. This at least represents a partial restoration of the medical act and the subject's choice faced with uncertainty.

In the *New York Times* article, Dr David A. Freedman, a clinical trials expert at the University of California, Berkeley, concludes with a snappy rhetorical formula: "We have machinery to pull diamonds from the earth, but we don't have machinery to pull truth from data in these studies." It couldn't be put any better. The clinical-studies machinery that is being applied to the field of psychotherapies is much worse: it is a machine run amok. We can see how, in submitting to the Procrustean-bed procedures that these studies enforce, the advocates of measurement have become prisoner to a course of study that is losing its head. The waves produced by these studies on the suicidogenic effect of antidepressants provide ample opportunity to observe that in the US and the UK, just as in France, the management of mental suffering by means of the ideology of evaluation is wearing thin. The ethical choice that a subject makes when he engages in a psychoanalysis or a relational psychotherapy, resorting at certain moments, if need be, to a drug therapy, has no reason to be short-circuited in the name of repetitive measurements of the effectiveness of standardised and pre-formatted techniques that have been drained of any substance. The procedurisation of the clinic has ushered in a stream of minor techniques that have been presented as "psychotherapies", but this is simply the peddling of defective stock that ought to be inspected with the same care that major brand names dedicate to stamping out industrial counterfeits.

Notes

1. The "Dodo Bird Verdict" is considered at greater length in the following chapter.
2. Colloquium of 20 March 2004 organised by C. Vasseur at Marly-le-roi. See the report by Agnès Aflalo at: http://www.oedipe.org/forum/read.php?6,1364.
3. The author cites Kendell & Jablensky, 2003.
4. [In the event, the DSM-5 was published on 22 May 2013. See the epilogue to this book. (Tr.)].
5. Also marketed under the brand names Vioxx, Ceoxx, and Ceeoxx.
6. Also marketed under the brand names Celebrex, Celebra, and Onsenal.
7. See too the chronicle of the ensuing months in Aflalo, 2014.
8. Also marketed under the brand names Aropax, Paxil, Pexeva, Seroxat, and Sereupin.
9. Anne Castot is in charge of scientific information at the French Agency for the Safety of Health Products (AFSSaPS).

CHAPTER FOUR

The psychopathy of evaluation

Originally published as "Blog-notes: psychopathie de l'évaluation" in La Cause freudienne, *issue 62, March 2006, pp. 51–70.**

The redefinition of the legal fiction *habeas corpus* by the healthcare systems has established a new healthcare policy: *not only is my body a legal fiction, now it has to be in good health as well*. The healthcare field used to be managed, from the ethical standpoint, by communities of medical professionals. So it remained for a long time, but economic concerns brought managerial administrative control to the fore, pushing professional ethics into the background. In the twenty-first century, the managerial formula has been implemented across the board: funding agencies, competitive tendering and sourcing, and the constitution of a market that is regulated to a greater or lesser extent by private-sector plans (the Health Maintenance Organisations in the US) or public-sector schemes (the UK and continental Europe system), all of which is shot through with the rhetoric of evaluation. The seeming

---

*This article was previously translated into English by Michelle Julien as "Blog-Notes: The Psychopathy of Evaluation" in the *Psychoanalytical Notebooks of the London Society,* issue 16, May 2007, pp. 45–75.

homogeneity of these solutions actually conceals a broad heterogeneity in the performance of the healthcare systems.

The American economist Paul Krugman has become an effective critic of the so-called "advantages" of privatisation. Highlighting the calamitous performance of the US healthcare system as a result of the deep imbalance in the privatisation of funding in the healthcare field, which effectively makes access to health care "a privilege rather than a right", he underscores how "this attitude turns out to be inefficient as well as cruel" (Krugman, 2005).[1] This has given rise to "agents" of the healthcare market who pass around "clients" who find themselves in a position of weakness, and this is happening at a time when healthcare systems are having to cope with a spectacular rise in demand for care which is linked not only to the fact of having a body but also to the fact of having a mind: *habeas mentem*.

Keeping one's psyche in good health is an imperative that is under-lined by the World Health Organization:

> The WHO [...] has drawn attention to the rise in demand for treat-ment of mental problems. One in four people have to cope with serious mental or psychiatric disturbances in the course of their existence and depressive disorders are set to become the most sig-nificant illness of the twenty-first century. (Pelc et al., 2005, p. 6)[2]

Faced with the explosion in demand for mental healthcare, the WHO is the bearer of good news. Following the example of somatic treatments whose effectiveness has been proven in keeping with the models of evidence-based medicine, the psychotherapies now fall within this same domain of proof. The psychotherapies, which constitute a spe-cific mode of treatment, are therefore being recognised scientifically as an effective treatment. Let's be quite clear on this point: nothing new has been invented. They have simply managed to make the psycho-therapies fit into the rhetoric of managerial evaluation by saying, for example:

> Encouraging evidence has recently emerged in relation to the cost-effectiveness of psychotherapeutic approaches to the management of psychosis and a range of mood and stress-related disorders, in combination with or as an alternative to pharmacotherapy. A consistent research finding is that psychological interventions lead to improved satisfaction and treatment concordance, which

can contribute significantly to reduced rates of relapse, fewer hospitalisations and decreased unemployment. The additional costs of psychological treatments are countered by decreased levels of other health service support or contact. (Murthy, 2001, p. 62; quoted in Perc et al., 2005, p. 6)

As we can see, the WHO is not sentimental. They plead compassionately for the psychotherapies in the name of a neo-liberal stance. The field of the psychotherapies is shared out into diverse orientations: psychoanalytic, cognitive-behavioural, systemic and relational. Though they do encourage the use of psychotherapies, the choice of modality is left to individual taste. From the managerial point of view, the question of choosing between psychotherapies is reduced to the question of their evaluation and their utility. Each of the different methods of evaluation start off from a limit that is met when measuring the effectiveness of the said psychotherapies: this limit sometimes goes by the name of the "Dodo Bird Verdict".

The problem of the Dodo Bird Verdict and the RCT power grab

The recent report from Belgium's Conseil supérieur d'Hygiène, which was compiled with the aim of enabling a psychotherapy bill to be drafted, sets out the problem as follows:

> The basic reference text, *Bergin and Garfield's Handbook of Psychotherapy and Behaviour Change* (Lambert, 2004), now in its fifth edition, offers a snapshot of the full range of empirical studies undertaken over the last sixty years. It emerges that psychotherapy is effective and enjoys *effect sizes* that are, on average, equivalent to those of somatic and medical treatments. In general, there is little or no difference when compared with the serious therapies (the famous "Dodo Bird Verdict", cf. Luborsky et al.), especially subsequent to rectifications carried out with the goal of taking into account the allegiance of the main researcher. The inter-personal processes (such as the building of a working alliance), and the person and expertise of the therapist (regardless of the orientation to which he adheres), turn out to have greater impact on variation in the effects than the specific techniques being used. (Pelc et al., 2005, pp. 15–16)[3]

The debate on the Dodo Bird Verdict is some thirty years old. The term is in homage to Lewis Carroll. In the second chapter of *Alice's Adventures in Wonderland*, Alice shrinks and finds herself in the pool of tears that she had wept when she was nine feet high. A mouse slips in too, then various other animals: "there were a Duck and a Dodo, a Lory and an Eaglet, and several other curious creatures" (Carroll, 1865, Ch. II). This troupe of animals is actually a re-casting of characters from Carroll's life. In Duck, one can identify the name of an old school friend, Robinson Duckworth, in Lory and Eaglet, the names of Alice's sisters, Lorina and Edith Lidell, and in Dodo, the actual surname of the author himself: Dodgson. It should be noted that the dodo is an extinct animal, that *Alice's Adventures in Wonderland* was first published in 1865, and that Darwin's *On the Origin of the Species* came out in 1859. The dodo, a Darwinian homage, is an emblematic animal from the Island of Mauritius that died out sometime around 1680, a victim of evolution. This name without reference denotes it in *Alice's Adventures in Wonderland* as the one who decides on the prizes following an open competition to find out how to get dry again. The mouse had proposed a semantic procedure, a story, "the driest thing I know", and now the dodo is proposing an asemantic procedure, "a Caucus-race", but no one knows what that is. Each of them interprets it in their own way and starts to run.

> When they had been running half an hour or so, and were quite dry again, the Dodo suddenly called out "The race is over!" [...] "But who has won?" [...] "*EVERYBODY* has won, and all must have prizes". (Carroll, 1865, Ch. III)

To arrive at this brilliant solution, the Dodo had to think long and hard: "it sat for a long time with one finger pressed upon its forehead (the position in which you usually see Shakespeare, in the pictures of him), while the rest waited in silence." His thinking betrayed no melancholia. This elegant solution to a test whose exact content is unknown to each of the participants, in which information is unequally and asymmetrically distributed, but from which each of them emerges as a winner, anticipates the formulation of a problem that was to occupy logicians and mathematicians in the next century.

Is there such a thing as a game with no losers, that is, a non-zero-sum game, which can be formulated mathematically? John Nash solved this question at the end of the 1950s. The "Nash equilibriums" designate possible economic games with a non-zero sum: all the participants come out winning. Might there be a similar kind of phenomenon in *bona fide* therapies? When they are measured, their effectiveness turns out to be more or less equivalent.

> Broadly speaking, most of the studies, meta-analyses and meta-meta-analyses indicate that there are few differences in the results obtained by so-called *bona fide* psychotherapies, that is, therapies that are guided by a coherent theoretical structure, which have been widely practised for a long time, and which have foundations for research [...] as is the case for cognitive-behavioural, systemic, psychoanalytic or [relational] psychotherapies. (Pelc et al., 2005, pp. 18–19 & p. 45)[4]

It was the will, the *hubris*, to go beyond this limit that marked out the 2004 Inserm collective report as an astonishing anomaly. This is how it has been singled out in the Belgian report:

> One remarkable exception is the recent Inserm report (2004) which presents itself as the first ever comparative research study to show the superiority of the cognitive-behavioural therapies over the other psychotherapies (except in the case of personality disorders). However, the methodological biases that led to these results have been widely noted [...]. (Pelc et al., 2005, p. 45)

They have, but not sufficiently so. Two years after the Inserm power grab which was followed by two further collective reports on the "psychological post-mortem of suicide" and "conduct disorder in children and adolescents", we now have a better understanding of what was going on. It occurred to a group of scientists that the only way to force a way out of the problem of the Dodo Bird Verdict was to employ a very particular method modelled on the randomised clinical trials (RCTs) used in the regulation of therapeutic goods.

To do so, they had to insist upon equivalence between psychotherapy and medication, this being the only way to justify drafting-in this method. As one of the experts, an advocate of CBT, puts it:

> Since the 1980s, the third generation of research in psychotherapy has been using the model of controlled clinical trials imported

from pharmacotherapy, along with DSM diagnostics and handbooks describing precisely which treatments to use. (Inserm, 2004, p. 44)

More than being a "third generation", this is a particular way of going about things, and a biased one at that. Let's take a closer look at these multiple biases.

When it comes to drug trials, the method consists in first obtaining perfectly homogenous groups of patients in conformity with a biological model that defines the cause of the illness. Next, the patients are shared out at random in accordance with an extremely standardised protocol, administering each patient *either* with strictly defined doses of the medicine to be tested *or* with a placebo or "reference" treatment. The prescriber does not know what he is prescribing. Invented as a way of restricting the pharmaceutical industry, the method now looks to be a machine running at full tilt as far as its applications for licences for psychotropic drugs are concerned, but is typified by the absence of any established biological causality for mental illnesses. Indeed, Philippe Pignarre has underlined how

> the biology of biochemical receptors in the brain [...] pushes to its triumphant conclusion the fact that a modern drug is invariably the next-to-latest one. There will always be another one that is more effective, more manageable, and less toxic. This "minor biology" gladly decks itself out in the trimmings of biology *per se*, but its ambitions are limited to the development of new drugs that will always be next-to-latest. (Pignarre, 2001, pp. 81–82)

One British psychiatrist has written with even greater precision on the absence of the biological model in psychiatry, pointing out that the dopaminergic "model" amounts to a reasoning along the lines of: aspirin brings relief to headaches, so headaches are caused by a deficit of acetylsalicylic acid (Rose, 2005, p. 28).

The interpretation of the results from the RCTs on the disinhibitory effects of antidepressants in teenagers has given rise to controversies, scandals and prescription bans. This is why the results of a study sponsored by a national organisation as opposed to a laboratory—the National Institute of Mental Health (NIMH) in the US—were awaited with special eagerness.[5] Now, the results of this study, which compares treatment by psychotherapy and/or Prozac in depressed teenagers, are paradoxical. On the one hand, they reassure doctors who were in fear of malpractice lawsuits: showing that pharmacotherapy alone had been effective in over 60% of cases proves that their prescription had been effective as well. On the other hand, the study lays ruin to the hopes generated by expert reports such as the Inserm study. In effect, cognitive-behavioural therapy, presented as a "psychotherapy" and a "talking therapy", does not demonstrate any greater effectiveness than placebo treatment. Cognitive-behavioural therapy as a "psychotherapy" thus finds itself effectively discredited as a preventative treatment for suicide.

As soon as these results were published, a *New York Times* article offered an insight into the unease that was being felt by all concerned. How can patients and their parents be reassured? How can they be helped to choose between the risks presented by antidepressants and the ineffectiveness of the "psychotherapies" represented by CBT? They sought to reassure the parents of depressed teenagers by observing that the results were less discouraging than they might seem (Carey, 2004). After all, even though the results are not very significant, psychotherapy by CBT did have an effect on 43% of patients, which is slightly higher than the 35% of those who improved with the placebo. The American academics went into action. They put the statistical data in their place, arguing that they do not take into account individual variations and thus highlight how results actually depend much more on particular cases and therapists than on comprehensive statistics. In a word, here we meet again the good old Dodo Bird Verdict interpretation. Some suspect that teenagers are too susceptible to their emotions to have the auto-observational attitude that it takes for CBT: they submit less to the note-taking duties and continuous self-monitoring. So as to come to a close and provide some peace of mind, the article concludes that there should be regular interviews with the teenage patient, especially given the suicide risk.

It is in this context that we also have to set the disparity from one country to the next in the rules for the prescription of antidepressants—disparities that are not easily justified—and the difficulty of establishing good-practice guidelines that are supposed to resolve any contradiction. The reader might care to refer to Anne Castot's July 2004 interview with Guy Hugnet. In the UK, they had just banned the use of Paroxetine for under-eighteens,

> while in the US they ha[d] settled for a warning, without
> prohibiting its use. In France, this drug [was] contraindicated
> for under-fifteens, but authorised in older teenagers and adults.
> (Hugnet, 2004, p. 51)

The French Agency for the Safety of Health Products acknowledged
the fact and replied:

> In France, Paroxetine has always been contraindicated for under-
> fifteens. Upwards of sixteen years of age, the reference is the results
> for adults. At the European level, there is an imbalance. This is
> why the Brussels Commission should soon be bringing legislation
> into line across the European member states. [...] It will be recom-
> mended to avoid using Paroxetine for under-eighteens, but without
> an absolute ban. The choice should be left to the prescribing doctor.
> Depending on the benefit/risk assessment for any given patient,
> the doctor will be able to prescribe as a last resort if there is no other
> solution. (Hugnet, 2004, p. 51)

The debate on the safety of antidepressant use applies to adults as well
(Carey, 2005). A study by the University of Ottawa finds that the risk of
attempted suicide is almost double in patients taking antidepressants.
Two further studies from the UK find on the contrary that there is no
significant risk of increase in suicide. In the light of these contradictory results, where should we put our trust? The *British Medical Journal*, which published all three studies, appeals to the clinical judgement
of practitioners and to the utilitarian good sense of patients (Cipriani
et al., 2005, pp. 373–374). This at least represents a partial restoration of
the medical act and the subject's choice in the face of uncertainty. In the
New York Times article, Dr David A. Freedman, a clinical trials expert at
the University of California, Berkeley, concludes with a snappy rhetorical formula: "We have machinery to pull diamonds from the earth, but
we don't have machinery to pull truth from data in these studies." It
couldn't be put any better!

The measure of homogeneity and neo-utilitarian puerility

We are touching here on one of the modalities of the impasse of randomised controlled trials and their methodology, a methodology that

some have presented as a be-all and end-all. The reasons for this are not contingent, but necessary: *there's no point in waiting for the next study before setting about resolving the contradictions and bypassing clinical judgement through the application of a standard protocol.*

More profoundly still, it has been observed that the transposition from these methods to comparative studies (either comparing psychotherapies with each other or comparing psychotherapies with pharmacotherapy) comes up against three obstacles. The first obstacle is the impossibility of obtaining population groups that are strictly homogenous. The second obstacle is the arbitrary and random allocation of one type of psychotherapy or another in defiance of both the patient's expectations and any prior transference. Lastly, the third obstacle is the impossibility of obtaining a strict standardisation of psychotherapeutic treatment, which is now reduced to the application of a handbook.

The scientists are ready to do anything to remove these obstacles.

Firstly, in order to obtain homogenous populations, they are prepared to slice up and compartmentalise the clinic so as to obtain cases in which only "pure" disorders would remain. The collective expert report by Inserm pushed this method a very long way. It singled out fifteen compartmentalised disorders, without any consideration of the personality as a whole, only then to tack on a sixteenth category: "personality disorders". As if by chance, psychodynamic therapies turn out to be the most effective when the personality is taken into account. This artificial cut between isolated disorders and the personality as a whole, which is a sheer artefact of these measures, then allows for the success of CBT to be extolled in fifteen cases out of sixteen! This artefact may be qualified as a "mereological error" to the extent that it consists in singling out parts from a whole and then treating both part and whole as though they were strictly equivalent. They measure out fifteen small parts and then, from the whole, they form an extra part.

The second obstacle to transposing the method is in establishing a control group, or placebo group. Some have underlined how distributing at random a set of patients who are consulting for mental problems (into an experimental group, a control group, a waiting list group or a placebo group) represents a deontological aberration. As the Belgian report insists, "one can only be alarmed at this kind of technique" (Pelc et al., 2005, pp. 45–46).[6] Furthermore, what is a placebo group in a field like ours where the placebo effect is crucial? It has been established that 15% of patients will already be faring better after the initial telephone call to set a first appointment, prior to any meeting. Clearly, to allow this to happen the clinician has to consent to occupy the place of the subject-supposed-to-know rather than eagerly destroying this place through authoritarian randomisation.

The third obstacle concerns the effect of exclusion produced on consulting patients as a whole by the standardisation of RCT. This effect is criticised in particular in a long article published in 2004 by three American authors who come to the following conclusion:

> Rather than focusing on treatment packages constructed in the laboratory designed to be transported to clinical practice and assuming that any single design (RCTs) can answer all clinically meaningful questions [...] we might do well to realign our goals [...]. (Westen et al., 2004, p. 658)[7]

Two other American authors, Ablon and Jones, summarise their criticisms as follows:

> Randomised clinical trials test a somewhat artificial treatment in an artificially controlled setting with atypical patients, so they have little generalisability to the real world of mental health care delivery. (Ablon & Jones, 2002, p. 775)

The limitations of the RCT method had already been revealed by the results of the NIMH Treatment of Depression Collaborative Research Program[8] which aimed to evaluate the effectiveness of CBT compared with "interpersonal therapy". This study, the results of which were published in the 1980s, produced a number of surprises. Firstly, it brought to light a comparable effectiveness for both of these two psychotherapies in the treatment of major depression, whilst drug therapy was only slightly more effective in the most severe cases. But this was not the surprise. The surprise came from the discrepancies in the results from the different study centres, despite the maximum possible standardisation of patients, therapists, and the manuals that they were supposed to be applying. How might these discrepancies be accounted for? The study was then supplemented by further refined measures and individual interviews which revealed that

> interpersonal psychotherapy conformed even more to the prototype of cognitive-behavioural therapy than to its own prototype.

In other words, the "interpersonal" therapists were doing CBT more than their own therapy and were obtaining better results than the cognitive-behavioural therapists doing CBT! (Thurin, 2005a)[9]

Thus, the disciples of CBT were taking an interest in processes of identification and the disciples of interpersonal therapy were not holding back their prescriptive advice. The discrepancies could not, therefore, be put down to either the therapies or the therapists. They depended on the subjects themselves, as to whether they were more or less "narcissistic". This was the variable that accounted most fully for the transferential effects and, therefore, for the therapeutic effects that were effectively obtained. Ultimately, the National Institute of Mental Health programme set out one of the major regularities that produce the Dodo Bird effect. In a framework as highly formatted as this one was (in view of the anticipation of evaluation), and in spite of the so-called "abstract" handbooks, the conformising effect is guaranteed. There you have it for what the Dodo Bird Verdict measures in large part.

All it takes then for this homogenisation to occur is for the measurement of rapid therapeutic effectiveness to be posited on the horizon at the outset. During a radio conversation, one psychoanalyst admitted that in many cases he did not shy away from accompanying the therapies he performs with something close to the kind of aversive exposure used in behavioural therapies. This is undoubtedly the uniformising effect that led to the Dodo Bird Verdict being hauled out again in Switzerland at the time of the debates on *Le Livre noir de la psychanalyse*. Professor of psychiatry and psychoanalyst Jean-Nicolas Despland, a specialist in the evaluation of psychotherapies, declared at the time:

> The results of psychoanalysis are hard to assess, and only very recently has it been playing the game of allowing itself to be assessed. But all the valid studies on the methodological plane show that in terms of effectiveness all schools have the same value. The type of therapy is ultimately a parameter of little importance for recovery. What is decisive is, on the one hand, the fact of letting the patient choose and, on the other, the quality of the therapist, whichever school he may belong to. (Arnal & Sibony, 2005, p. 24)

A conforming and homogenising effect can also be produced once the emulation of RCT methods (which are said to be "quantitative") starts to push towards the development of qualitative methods that would allow for the complexity of clinical reality to be taken into account. These qualitative methods have received a number of different names. The authors of the Belgian report recommend not trusting in the RCT results alone but rather taking into account other evaluative approaches (of which they single out four;[10] Pelc et al., 2005, p. 16). For example, the German Society of the International Psycho-Analytic Association (DPV) launched a "qualitative"[11] study to evaluate patients' retrospective appraisals of their psychoanalysis or psychoanalytic therapy and its effects, several years after the final session. Published in the *International Journal of Psycho-Analysis*, the results show the effectiveness of psychoanalytic treatment, both from the point of view of the patients—more than 70% of them reported positive changes across different registers[12]—and from the point of view of the symptomatology evaluation scales, because they "indicate that the majority of former patients are no longer disturbed to the point that they would still be diagnosed as clinically ill". The individual benefits are accompanied by a study of the utilitarian extensions for the good of one and all, and this is expressed in terms that are close to those of the WHO report:

> With regard to expenses in the healthcare sector, this study has shown that long-term therapies have helped to reduce costs in a permanent way in other medical disciplines. This fact was highlighted by the fewer number of days out of work and days of hospitalisation. Furthermore, costs also diminished indirectly, whether through heightened creativity and professional efficacy, or because patients who were previously unemployed found new jobs, or even because their capacity to react empathetically towards their own children was significantly increased, or because they overcame social isolation by getting involved in social and public engagements. (Pelc et al., 2005, p. 20)

As we can see, the full human dimension is taken into account in this utilitarianism that knows no bounds. Nothing is said in the study about their having drawn back the veil on the private lives of these patients, which is what the retroactive constitution of such lists entails. No question is raised as to the complete suspension of confidentiality that this implies and there is not the slightest questioning as to the eagerness to respond that these former patients demonstrated. We are looking here at the installation of a veritable panopticon, a kind of rash and fool-hardy imitation of the procedure of the Pass founded on getting people to speak about their analysis to researchers who are inspired by psycho-social methods.

The neo-utilitarian puerility of the research results thus obtained can be compared with the homogenising effect of the measurement meth-ods: everyone does the same thing and no one aims any higher. So it is that they obtain what Jacques-Alain Miller has called a "Panopticon [...] on the cheap" (Miller, 2006).

The effects of the eagerness to destroy the subject-supposed-to-know

Among these so-called "qualitative" evaluations, some are more interesting than others, for example, those that accentuate subjective preferences rather than the measurement of effects of conformity. The American Psychological Association seems to have noticed this. From 1995 on, the APA had been supporting RCT studies, but is now chang-ing its orientation towards other paths as is borne out by a draft policy statement by the 2005 presidential task force of the APA (see Thurin, 2005b).[13] The APA is seeking to sustain an approach that allows for the patient's treatment preferences to be taken into account, rather than depending on randomised authoritarian allocation. After having ceded to the sirens of evidence-based medicine, the APA is now insisting on the limitations of the false scientistic universal. Adapting to the particu-lar situation of each subject supposes taking into account each subject's expectations of his psychotherapy. One has to move from evidence-based evaluation to value-based evaluation. Authoritarian and ran-domised allocation introduces extra bias by flouting the values of each individual subject. There are those who wish to speak or to know some-thing about their symptom, and there are those who wish to be rid of a disturbance as though it were a foreign body, without wanting to know anything more about it. The decreed recommendations for treatment ought to be able to take this into account. As the authors of the Belgian report write, the decision the subject takes with regard to his treatment "always implies a complex process of evaluation which, even though it is 'science-informed', is also guided by [his] individual situation, [his] values and [his] wishes". These choices are therefore always "values-based", i.e. [based] on the value that each client ascribes to ethically acceptable personal preoccupations: for example, fewer symptoms and greater understanding of his mental functioning. (Pelc et al., 2005, p. 16)[14]

Behind this mask of value, on which no subject wants to cede, there lies concealed the supposition of knowledge that the subject attributes, or not, to the Other he addresses.

Beyond mental healthcare, other domains in the social field, which have already met the perverse effects of assessment techniques and evaluative rhetoric, are also perceiving the consequences of this eagerness to destroy the subject-supposed-to-know, an eagerness that is masked beneath the appearance of the necessity for transparency. The eagerness to see and expose every which procedure, every which way of doing, ends up crushing democratic debate and promoting the tyranny of the One. As Marilyn Strathern writes:

> In a social world where people are conscious of diverse interests, such an appeal to a benevolent or moral visibility is all too easily shown to have a tyrannous side—there is nothing innocent about making the invisible visible. (Strathern, 2000, p. 309)

In the UK, universities and research bodies in particular have suffered from the loss induced by what is claimed to be a "gain in evaluative information". More information comes at the cost of less trust and a blow to the social bond.

> This especially applies to expert systems, such as characterise the undertaking of scientific research or the teaching of students. Such practices cannot be made fully transparent simply because there is no substitute for the kind of experiential and implicit knowledge crucial to expertise, and which involves trust of the practitioners ("respect", Scott, 2000) and, we may add, among or between them ("tacit knowledge", Gibbons et al., 1994). On the contrary, the information society which promises to deliver "the ideal of transparency ... undermines the trust that is necessary for an expert system to function effectively" (Tsoukas, 1997, p. 835). (Strathern, 2000, p. 313)

We have only to replace this sociological use of the term "trust" with the specifically psychoanalytic term "transference" to uncover what pertains to we psychoanalysts in all this. When it is a matter of knowledge and transmission, the sociologists themselves discern the importance of *implicit knowledge*, of the subject-supposed-to-know, which is crucial for the implementation of transference as the basis of the experience.

After noting the destructive effects that the evaluation culture has been having on universities and research bodies, and even though some voices have been advising a "qualitative" counterculture of evaluation, we may wonder whether such a thing as "good assessment" is really possible. The authors of one collective book, coordinated by a social-sciences researcher at the University of Montreal, far from sharing the biopsychosocial conception of symptoms taught by their rival, McGill University (a chief purveyor of evaluative rhetoric), have insisted on the necessity of changing perspective. To do so, they have set them-selves "the objective of rethinking the notion and the mechanisms of evaluation for the quality of services in Quebec from the users' point of view" (Rodriguez Del Barrio et al., 2005, back cover). They lay the emphasis on the perverse effects that arise when care structures are standardised in accordance with strict protocols ruled by quantitative indicators. This becomes especially important as the care distribution systems become more concentrated. Moreover, it is underlined that the "complexity" of the problems encountered in the field of mental health necessitates a "plurality of perspectives and practices",[15] all the more so given that the protagonists are confronted with "work on the self [that] largely exceeds the control of symptoms". Pursuing this line of research on qualitative criteria, the authors of the book are then led to put for-ward indicators for quality.[16] But are there not grounds to fear that the effect produced by these indicators might ultimately lead to conformis-ing effects that are different but just as present?

Occupying a place on the political chessboard that is symmetrical to that of Marilyn Strathern, the liberal commentator David Brooks draws analogous conclusions on the pitfalls of evaluation as applied to edu-cation. Consider his criticism of the US education system for its vast evaluation programme justifying the Bush administration's No Child Left Behind Act of 2001.

> The stuff you can measure with tests is only the most superficial component of human capital. [...] No Child Left Behind treats students as skill-acquiring cogs in an economic wheel [...]. These

programmes are not designed for the way people are. The only
things that work are local, human-to-human immersions that transform the students down to their very beings. Extraordinary schools,
which create intense cultures of achievement, work. Extraordinary teachers, who inspire students to transform their lives, work.
(Brooks, 2005)

What Brooks here calls "local, human-to-human immersions" is his
formulation, in the neo-managerial language of the people he is address-
ing, of the non-eliminable character of the embodied subject-supposed-
to-know.

To summarise our criticisms of the results of evaluation we can say
that measurement, such as it is applied to psychotherapy, only takes
into account the most superficial aspects of the process in course, and
that it tends to conformise and homogenise all its elements. It does not
teach us anything about what really goes on. It is time to turn our backs
once and for all on this approach and its overriding tendency to produce standardised therapies for formatted disorders. We need to train
psychoanalysts who are capable of best applying psychoanalysis to the
patient who calls upon them, taking full account of the complexity of
the context of this appeal. We need, always, to discern in any given
situation its extraordinary character instead of trimming it down on the
Procrustean bed of a standardised protocol.

Evaluating ODD and the psychotherapies
under the scientistic gaze

The acts of violence that shook the French suburbs in November 2005
put on centre stage the eagerness of various different government
figures to promote the study of violent behaviour with an eye to deter-
mining preventative measures. Experts in biopolitical population management were summoned to calm the anxiety. Two documents, both
exemplary in their genre, were published at the time.

Consider first the collective expert report from Inserm, *Trouble des
conduites chez l'enfant et l'adolescent* [*Conduct Disorder in Children and
Adolescents*]. Here, "disorder" corresponds to a sociopathic definition
and pools together abundantly heterogeneous elements. It includes a
wide

palette of very diverse lines of behaviour that range from the temper tantrums and recurrent disobedience of difficult children to serious acts of aggression like rape, bodily harm, and delinquent theft. (Inserm, 2005, p. ix)[17]

Conduct disorder has been singled out as a "risk factor" for delinquency and its treatment would purportedly enable delinquency to be prevented. In this report, Inserm focuses once again on a flaw at the level of "biological equipment" which it views as requiring urgent measurement from the time each child is born. Refusal of social norms is imputed to cognitive deficits which can be measured by two—and only two—distinct functions. This refers to a Theory-of-Mind impairment in the subject that would entail, on the one hand, a failure to identify with others ("mind-blindness"), and on the other, a failure to inhibit action. These deficits are taken into account at the expense of any possibility of the clinical historicisation of symptoms; symptoms which have thereby been cut off from any singular articulation that bears a signifying dimension. The subject's history is then reduced to the role of merely favouring certain factors in the environment that influence gene-expression.

Of course, this "conduct disorder" does not stand alone, that is, without the notorious "associated disorders". For our experts this disorder ought not, however, to be too hastily linked to personality disorders. Indeed, in its clinical diversity, it is related first and foremost to hyperkinetic disorder with attention-deficit and to oppositional defiant disorder (ODD). From the perspective of a genetic flaw, one next has to measure comorbidity with other disturbances such as anxiety disorders, depressive disorders or learning difficulties, which are considered to be distinct and compartmentalised entities. Here again, they consider this comorbidity to be present since birth. No other therapeutics is envisaged by the experts besides educative supervision and the full arsenal of drugs that the psychiatrist has at his disposal: anti-psychotics, thymo-regulators, and psycho-stimulants.

The troubling prospect of seeing children's health records noted with such items as "fought/struck/bit/kicked/disobeyed/remorseless" upset a broad swathe of the public, far beyond the specialists. Columns in the daily papers filled with indignant reactions from a wide range of educators and other professionals. The international women's weekly

Elle also expressed alarm at this potential information logging on infants and young children.

In this respect, the public hearing *Prise en charge de la psychopathie* organised by the Haut Autorité de santé (HAS), which was opened to a fairly large audience of three hundred people on 15–16 December 2005, may be considered as a marketing exercise on the same subject, functioning as a flipside to the Inserm report. The wording of the title on its own holds great significance: instead of starting off from a loosely defined "disturbance", the hearing went under the banner "Taking Charge of Psychopathy". The term "psychopathy" belongs to our clinical tradition, even though it tends to be seldom used nowadays. Instead of asserting a willingness to replace the clinic with a knowledge that comes from statistical studies, the hearing saw practicing professionals auditioning papers that bore not only on biological studies but also on clinical studies. The bibliography that was provided was not restricted to Anglo-American statistical studies; it also included French articles of a psychoanalytic persuasion. A "bibliographical summary" presenting a digest of the cited works was drafted by the Marseilles-based psychiatrist Dr Sarfati, who had taken part in the *Forums des psys* organised in the wake of the Accoyer Amendment. Nonetheless, the limits of these open doors need to be noted: not one Lacanian analyst featured among the authors who were auditioned.

The intention of this collection is set out in its conclusion. It was a matter of duly taking note of a profession that was deeply divided

> between, on one hand, a biologising current, heir to the DSM, which diagnoses disorders without considering any links to the subject's history, and which privileges behavioural therapies (which draw on learning and conditioning theories), and, on the other, a psychodynamic current that acknowledges the contributions of psychoanalysis and uses them to tackle care as well as to tackle the modalities of its practices, and which considers each subject in his history and in his singularity. (HAS, 2005, p. 169)

This division is produced under the watchful eye of a master who is anything but divided.

For the HAS, the goal is clear: to develop an instrument that can be used by judges so that they will know how to punish and implement surveillance over the authors of violence: "It is likely that the psychiatric assessments requested by the judicial system will differ as to their content, depending on the psychiatrist's training and orientation" (HAS, 2005, p. 169). In this sense, the different contributions are conceived of as a *vade mecum* for magistrates, and the utilitarian intention is writ large.

In the future, the evaluation scale will supplant clinical acumen in the practice of psychiatry. The path to objectification and the exit from this question of the clinical field is traced out by François Caroli in his introduction to the hearing: "The difficulty of tackling psychopathy resides in the fact that it combines in its very description 'social semiology' and 'clinical semiology'", with one bound to the other (Caroli, 2005, p. 14). The term "psychopathy" is a product of "different times and cultures, creating a multitude of nosographic concepts". Then, "faced with this polymorphism which is hard to describe, a whole system of dismemberment progressively fell into place for a kind of objectivity, indeed a kind of objectification, through the [suppression] of the term 'psychopath'" from the APA classification of mental illnesses (Caroli, 2005, p. 14).[18] As Caroli observes,

> the oddest thing (and on this point only the notion of "hysteria" has suffered the same fate) resides in the fact that having completely disappeared from the nomenclature, it nonetheless remains an extremely pertinent element when it comes to describing certain present-day clinical realities.

Likewise, whilst the DSM clinic is criticised by those psychologists and sociologists who do not hum the same tune as those of a biological persuasion, they do stress its omnipresence. Serge Lesourd, professor of psychology at Strasbourg, gives a wry presentation of the cultural dimension of ODD. Here, first of all, are the opening diagnostic criteria as listed in the DSM:

> Negativistic, hostile and defiant behaviour [for] at least six months [including at least four of the following criteria]: often loses temper; often argues with adults; often actively defies or refuses to comply with adults' requests or rules; often deliberately annoys people; often blames others for his or her mistakes or misbehaviour; is often touchy or easily annoyed by others; is often angry and resentful; is often spiteful or vindictive. (APA, 1995)

Lesourd comments on the effect produced by the senselessness of these items:

> The reading that the DSM-IV offers of ODD includes a dubious aspect because turning "opposition" into "disorder" effaces any possibility of grasping the meaning of a rebellion, a meaning which is sometimes justified. If we consider the reading of this same adolescent disorder by drawing on a social reading of the same signs, we would get what in 1970 was the definition of "the Leftist", and in 2000 the definition of "the struggling youth". If we employ a political reading, then we would be looking in 1970 at a "troublemaker" and in the 2000s at a "wild child". If we read these signs in the light of psychoanalytic theory, we might be able to speak in terms of "narcissistic personality" or "borderline". [...] The psychopathies should thus be understood as a social symptom; they are constructed within the coordinates of the social moment at which the impasses of the subject are met. (Lesourd, 2005, p. 17)

Likewise, child psychiatrists have pointed up contradictions in the ICD-10 and DSM definitions of anti-social personality. The DSM specifies that the diagnosis can only be made if the patient is "at least 18 years old [and has] had symptoms of conduct disorder before age 15". Drs Marcelli and Cohen highlight how this

> short sentence, which has been included somewhat surreptitiously, in actual fact poses extremely complex questions. If one accepts the ideology of the DSM-IV with respect to the categorising of the disorders described, a point of view which rejects any dimensional aspect but also any developmental aspect, how is this sudden age-dependent change of category to be understood? Can an illness befall an individual simply because he turns eighteen? (Marcelli & Cohen, 2005, p. 25)

On the other hand, pointing out the quandary that the category of ODD gives rise to for the ICD-10 itself—indeed the handbook specifies that this "category is included to reflect common diagnostic practice and to facilitate the classification of disorders occurring in young children"[19]—Marcelli and Cohen conclude: "One sometimes has the impression that the ICD-10 looks for excuses for having introduced this disorder in this way with such imprecise contours!" (Marcelli & Cohen, 2005, p. 29).

The same authors also offer a critique of the very notion of comorbidity in the medical model:

> Comorbidity is a major problem in the diagnosis of Attention-Deficit Hyperactivity Disorder in children, adolescents or even adults. It is extremely complicated to dissociate the combined effects of ADHD from true comorbidities. (Marcelli & Cohen, 2005, p. 29)[20]

Everything is localised in the articulation between the morbid and the comorbid. But where does the crux of the matter really lie?

Lastly, far from sharing Inserm's enthusiasm for the cognitive causality of the disorder, Marcelli and Cohen underline that the "neuro-radiologic, neuropsychological and neuro-endocrinian explorations (the genetic studies) have not, despite their number, yielded significant results" and ADHD refers to an aetiology that is still unknown (Marcelli & Cohen, 2005, p. 27).[21]

These critical viewpoints merely highlight, however, the far-reaching invasion of the *biologising* conception. Thus we see Thierry Pham showing great enthusiasm for the Hare checklist, which allows for the ideal psychopath to be singled out from the category of antisocial personalities (Pham, 2005, pp. 31–32). According to Pham, the distinction obtained by employing rating scales such as these would serve to predict not only the subject's type of violence (violent robbery rather than sex offences or murder) but also his likelihood of re-offending. Lastly, the tautology which holds that psychopathic behaviour is poorly controlled behaviour serves to found this clinical category which is not easily supported by any clear-cut genetic deficiency: "psychopathy might be the result of a neuro-developmental disorder linked to affects" (Pham, 2005, p. 32). Emotional deficiency—the psychopath's coldness—would thus be explained by lesions in the frontal cortex or dysfunction in the amygdala. Here we meet once again the *continuum* that we have already noted in the hypotheses of the Inserm experts on conduct disorder in children. We can see that glandular deficiencies are going to be an increasingly common reference point.[22] From phobics to psychopaths, disturbances in the functioning of the amygdala are going to be asked to explain a great deal.

The true function of Inserm's extremist stance is perhaps not to convince the profession as a whole, but rather to accustom it to radical formulations, to positions on the scientist front line, and to biologising ritornellos. Once the habit has been instilled, the Haut Autorité de santé will have only to present itself as a conciliator so as to have the rank and file swallow the pill of this would-be "modernist" line and maintain a supposed equilibrium. Whether the manoeuvre will succeed cannot be certain given the scale of the problem, for example, when psychopathic conduct alternates with out-and-out psychotic manifestations (see Zagury, 2005).

www.psychopaths.ue

Beyond the scales and checklists, can there be such a thing as a like-able psychopath? If there is one who might be able to stake a claim to this title, it would be Frank Abagnale Jr. The book that Abagnale wrote on his life as a psychopath was turned into a feature film by Steven Spielberg in 2002 (Spielberg, 2002). The film portrays him as a cool con man, a narcissistic seducer, an expert counterfeiter of forged checks under numerous false names, and an antihero in a family spectacle. Leonardo Di Caprio plays in turn a young man, a doctor, a lawyer and, above all, a pilot. This was the era when these professions were seen as the acme of "sexy" as far as serious virility goes. Back then, airline travel was not the security-conscious obstacle course that it is today. Pilots had "the right stuff" and air hostesses were real supermodels. Frank's father is presented as being about as undependable as John le Carré's—which is no small matter—and his mother as a narcissistic woman who is distant and irresponsible. Moreover, there is an aggravating circumstance from the moral standpoint: she is French. From this formidable cocktail, Spielberg succeeds in weaving an unsettling spectacle that wends its way through complete misunderstanding. The New York Times critic Stephen Holden couldn't resist calling it, "the most charming of Mr Spielberg's mature films" (Holden, 2002).

One could say that Frank Abagnale is not a psychopath but a mythomaniac who has been pacified by prison life and by the neo-paternal obstinacy of his pursuer, or even that he would have a very low score on the Hare checklist, and so on. Very well, but this does not change the fascination that is compelled by the cold narcissism of the psychopath whose action falls wide of the comprehensible motivations of neurosis or the reactions of substantiated psychosis and cruel perversions.

What question does he put to us? For us, the clinic of the symptom, taken as a whole, is divided into the signifying face of its formal envelope and the libidinal charge of the object *a*. These two faces are linked as are the two faces of a Möbius strip. One can say that these two dimensions hold together by the bond of the *sinthome*. Truth and jouissance are thus taken up in a continuous fabric. The dimension of the sinthome that is approached by psychoanalytic experience denotes what Jacques-Alain Miller has called "a real for psychoanalysis" (Miller, 1997). This real does not obey any law. On the contrary, it denotes what forms an obstacle to the *parlêtre* being regulated in any way. The de-regulating that is situated by the "psychopathic" entity is a case that lies on the borderline. He is a subject who obeys nothing. He is a residual figure where jouissance and norms tie in with one another without any transcendence and without any call upon prohibition.

According to Lacan, this real which psychoanalysis deals with vouches for the omnipresence of jouissance in the Other. The fascination with the psychopath's actions is founded on the idea of a being who would be "jouissance through and through". He would thus have broken off from the signifier in a way that is different from, though just as effective as, that of the autist, a case that lies on the borderline of the field of psychosis. In actual fact, the "ideal" psychopath repeats actions that never lead to an act. These actions testify to the missed encounter with the trauma of language.

The psychopath acts in such a way that he ignores prohibition and the dialectic that binds prohibition to transgression. He nonetheless reminds us, in his own way, how the central question for the *parlêtre* is that of the place of jouissance which prohibition merely indicates. Lacan does not formulate prohibition without jouissance. Prohibition protects us from the jouissance that causes anxiety. This is why, in his "Discours aux Catholiques", he approaches *Totem and Taboo* from the angle of anxiety and jouissance:

> Freud's reflection in *Totem and Taboo* revolves around the function of the phobic object, and it is this function that puts him on the road to the Father function. Indeed, this latter function constitutes a turning point between the preservation of desire [...] and the correlative principle of a prohibition that bears on the sidelining of this

desire. These two principles wax and wane together, though their effects are different—the omnipotence of desire generating the fear of the defence that ensues in the subject, prohibition chasing out from the subject his *statement* of desire so as to make it pass over into an Other, into this unconscious that knows nothing of what its *enunciation* supports. (Lacan, 2005b, p. 35)

By laying the emphasis on jouissance, Lacan comes to set out this nexus in a different way. Jouissance becomes the first factor. The superego says *Jouis!* ["Enjoy!"] and the Other's signifiers turn out to be implicated because the subject replies *J'ouïs!* ["I hear!"]. The parasite of language, which is the Other as such, traumatises the body, it gives rise to the *parlêtre*'s jouissance and the encounter therewith in the symptom or sinthome.

The psychopath is the nether side of the sinthome. Far from being a saint, he is rather the damned of the symptom, but he motions in its direction. For us, the comorbidity of ODD, ADHD, GAD and other BPDs motion towards RSI, SIR, IRS and towards the Name-of-the-Father as an instrument. These letters name the different modes by which the real, the symbolic and the imaginary tie in, modes by which we endeavour to think through the symptom in its particularity. The traumatic impact of the language parasite on the living being produces the sinthome, the stem cell that allows for the language parasite to be grafted onto the body and for the *parlêtre* to be produced.

Our world is no longer lived as something that is dominated by a transcendent prohibition. Transcendence is no longer the transcendence of divine prohibition, which it is so difficult to maintain now that science has silenced its voices. Science and The Divine are, however, henceforth linked in a different way. What now holds the place of truth is scientific certainty as to the world's objectivity. Eternal truths have stepped aside in favour of "objective truths", but God still lurks here. Willard Van Orman Quine concluded his excellent 1953 article "Two Dogmas of Empiricism" with the statement of his private and ironic religion. He gives the God of philosophers and scientists a momentous twist:

> For my part I do, qua lay physicist, believe in physical objects and not in Homer's gods; and I consider it a scientific error to believe otherwise. But in point of epistemological footing the physical

objects and the gods differ only in degree and not in kind. Both
sorts of entities enter our conception only as cultural posits. The
myth of physical objects is epistemologically superior to most in
that it has proved more efficacious than other myths as a device for
working a manageable structure into the flux of experience. (Quine,
1953, p. 44, §II, 6)

These objects, these gods, denote a real that lies outside language.
Richard Rorty's pragmatism goes further still, standing in opposition
to any meta-language conception of truth. For Quine, scientific laws
are those that support an "objective" real. This is the dimension outside
language that enables science to hold firm through its very impossibility of absorbing the real. For Rorty, there is no longer any impossible
point outside language. This is why his colleague Simon Blackburn has
criticised pragmatism for its *levelling* side, obtained by considering only
the utility of language games. Here is how Rorty reports on the debate:

Blackburn writes that pragmatism is characterised by "the denial
of differences, the celebration of the seamless web of language, the
soothing away of distinctions, whether of primary versus second-
ary qualities, fact versus value, description versus expression, or of
any other significant kind. What is left is a smooth, undifferentiated
view of language." Blackburn goes on to say that this view may easily lead to "minimalism, deflationism, or quietism." This is exactly
what I take language to be like. (Engel & Rorty, 2007, p. 33)[23]

Replace pragmatic utilitarianism with the satisfaction of jouissance and
we get a quietism of jouissance. In the dimension of the other real, the
lawless real, the psychopath, through his mad, deregulated, repetitive,
senseless, and untreatable action recalls for us the presence of the primordial world prior to any prohibition. The continuous fabric of language and jouissance does not authorise quietism. The psychopath
strives to produce a tear in this fabric through the short-circuit of his
action. The enigma of his way of proceeding hangs over the circle of the
violent damned. This enigma holds many more questions in store for
us. One can full well imagine the next step for the HAS audition process: the creation of a website. We recommend registering it under the
domain name ".ue". *Allez, hue!* Giddy up! It will take another effort to
free the studies on psychopathy from the straitjacket of the checklist.

Notes

1. See also McKibbin, 2006, pp. 3–6.
2. Here the authors are referring to reports published by the WHO in 2001, 2002, 2003, and 2005.
3. See also: Luborsky et al., 2002; Lambert, 2003; Norcross, 2002; Wampold, 2001.
4. See also: Messer, 2002; Smith & Glass, 1977; Shapiro & Shapiro, 1982; Shapiro & Shapiro, 1983; Wampold et al., 1997; Grissom, 1996; Luborsky, 2002; Wampold, 2001.
5. The first results of this study were presented in June 2004; cf., March et al., 2004.
6. The authors also cite Roger Perron et al. (2004): "How can anyone, if indeed there are such people, who applies himself in this way *not* to treat, believe himself and call himself a 'psychotherapist'? How can one deliberately lie to people who are suffering and asking for help?"
7. Here we reproduce a part of their conclusions:

> The average RCT for most disorders currently described as empirically supported excludes between one third and two thirds of patients who present for treatment, and the kinds of patients excluded often appear both more representative and more treatment resistant in naturalistic studies. For most disorders, particularly those involving generalised symptoms such as major depression or GAD [general anxiety disorder], brief, largely cognitive-behavioural treatments have demonstrated considerable efficacy in reducing immediate symptomatology. The average patient for most disorders does not, however, recover and stay recovered at clinically meaningful follow-up intervals. [...] Despite frequent claims in the literature about treatment of choice, few data are available comparing manualised treatments with treatment as usual [...]. What is known is that treatments in the community tend to be substantially longer than treatments in the laboratory, regardless of the therapist's theoretical orientation, and that in naturalistic samples, more extensive treatments tend to achieve better results according to both patient and clinician reports.

Note that the term "naturalistic studies" refers to studies conducted in ordinary care structures and not in clinical "research laboratories" on artificially complicit populations. This homage to "nature" is somewhat curious here. Perhaps the cultural dimension of the clinic is being denied.

8. Jean-Michel Thurin describes the collaborative research programme on the treatment of depression as follows:

> launched in the mid-eighties [and supported by the] National Institute of Mental Health, [the programme sought] to test the effectiveness of two forms of short-term psychotherapy in the out-patient treatment of (non-bipolar and non-psychotic) depressed patients who corresponded to the diagnosis of Major Depressive Disorder. The two therapies, the effectiveness of which had been partially shown in previous studies, were the cognitive-behavioural therapy developed by Beck et al. at the University of Pennsylvania and the interpersonal psychotherapy described by Klerman, Weissman et al. in New Haven and Boston. (Thurin, 2005)

9. J.-M. Thurin concludes: "in actual fact, what are habitually termed 'non-specific effects' could very well be the coexistence in different therapies of specific technical factors: equivalent processes give equivalent results."

10. "[i] open clinical trials in natural contexts—admittedly without a control group, but with greater external validity; [ii] research into the effects of the processes, in which the links between certain process variables and (intermediary) effects are investigated; [iii] multiple 'case design', during the course of which the development of the process can be analysed in depth; and [iv] in-depth research on the specific procedures and processes of change."

11. The first stage in this research was to obtain the agreement of the psychoanalysts, who came out 89% in favour of the study. The second stage was to determine a representative sample of all the patients in long-term psychoanalytic treatment that had ended during a period determined by the study; this stage did not pose any recruitment problems either ($n = 401$). The material was multiform: recorded interviews with open or semi-open questionnaires. The interviews (two for each former patient, to which was added a third with the former analyst) were recorded and studied with the researchers. (Leuzinger-Bohleber et al., 2003).

12. Here is what the Conseil Supérieur d'Hygiène reports on this point (Pelc et al., 2005, p. 19): "In their questionnaires, 75% of patients retrospectively qualified their general state as 'poor' prior to psychotherapy and 81% qualified their general state as 'good' after psychotherapy; 80% of patients mentioned positive changes during long-term treatment with respect to their mental condition, their inner growth, and their

relational life; between 70 and 80% indicated positive changes with respect to their capacity to cope with life events, their self-esteem and mood, as well as their satisfaction with their lives and their efficiency."

13. Thurin cites the "2005 Presidential Task Force on Evidence-Based Practice: Draft Policy Statement on Evidence-Based Practice in Psychology" 25 February 2005 (available online at http://forms.apa.org/members/ebp/ebp.pdf).

14. Here the authors are referring to Fulford et al., 2004.

15. They write: "The complexity of these problems meets a margin of uncertainty and should encourage us to maintain an open space of experimentation and evaluation of different practices using pluralistic criteria and viewpoints, including: the perspectives of the biological sciences and human sciences; the perspectives of mental health workers, users, and their close ones; and regional specificity and the way other cultures understand and approach these problems. Maintaining a plurality of perspectives and practices seems here to be essential to the advancement of knowledge and to the hope of a better life for the chief protagonists. Serious mental health problems are generally accompanied by deep existential questioning for the people who have to live with these problems." (Rodriguez Del Barrio et al., 2001, p. 220).

16. The frame in which the authors situate themselves "offers criteria and indicators of quality that will allow for the evaluation of results, practices, and the organisation of services in the community as well as the institutional mechanisms that are necessary to guarantee its application and to ensure quality service performance. This particularly concerns the mental health sector, but introduces considerations and a model of reflection that [can] be [applied] to many other domains of healthcare and social services." (Rodriguez Del Barrio et al., 2005)

17. See in particular: Laurent, 2005; Misès, 2005.

18. Caroli specifies that this disappearance "follows on directly from the work of Cleckley (1941) who, in *The Mask of Sanity*, finds the word 'psychopathy' to be a stigmatising one".

19. Entry F91.3: Oppositional Defiant Disorder (WHO, 1994, p. 212).

20. Marcelli and Cohen note that, "the literature identifies with certainty three types of comorbidity: externalised disorders (ODD and CD) in 40 to 90% of ADHD subjects; internalised disorders (anxiety, depression) in 25 to 40% of ADHD subjects; and learning difficulties in 10 to 92% of ADHD subjects [...]. Comorbidity with internalised disorders is purportedly more frequent in children who present inattention-dominant ADHD whilst in children who present hyperactivity/impulsivity-dominant ADHD (or mixed forms) comorbidity with externalised disorders appears more often." (Marcelli & Cohen, 2005, p. 27)

21. "Several computerised tests are available for assessing Attention Deficit, notably in [its] two dimensions of selective attention and general attention. [...] To this day, the aetiology of ADHD remains unknown and diagnosis depends on the full set of clinical elements gathered from the parents, the child, and close adults (teachers), on the careful study of antecedents, and on a comparison of (neurological, cognitive, neuropsychological and language proficiency) assessment reports." (Marcelli & Cohen, 2005, p. 27)

22. The amygdalian model of the psychopath conflicts with other models. For example, the *Economist* article "The Omega Point" (2006a, p. 72) reports research on foetal metabolism and Omega-3 acids implied in the regulation of serotonin: low levels during pregnancy purportedly result in "pathological social interactions", in an "inability to make friends", and later in "aberrant behaviour". Whether the model is serotonergic or amygdalian, the psychopath is deemed to have been that way from the very start.

23. Rorty is citing Blackburn, 1998, p. 157.

PART III

PSYCHOANALYSIS AND COGNITION

CHAPTER FIVE

On the origin of the Other
and the post-traumatic object

The following lecture was delivered at the Institut des Sciences Cognitives in Lyon on 6 November 2004 and was later published as "L'origine de l'Autre et l'objet post-traumatique" in the Bulletin de l'ACF Rhône-Alpes, issue 88/89, November 2006.

I would like to thank the organisers of this conference for providing me with the opportunity to delight with you in defying a prohibition, one that was laid down by the French Society of Linguistics in 1886 and which pertains to the origin of tongues, the very same prohibition of which Éric Saïer has shown us a facsimile,[1] knowing full well the indubitable adaptive advantage I would draw from it.

Jakobson's structuralism respected this watchword. Linguistics still harboured the memory of the cumbrous debate on the origin of tongues, which compared the respective ages of Greek, Latin, and Hebrew, and the search for the perfect language, the Abrahamic tongue (see Eco, 1995; Milner, 2002). Only the refusal of this problematic paved the way for the success of the comparative grammar of the Indo-European languages.

Likewise, the question of the origin of civilisations and their classification in terms of evolution (measured in relation to their supposed starting-point) encumbered ethnological thought with a certain quantity of dross, for example, the notorious myth of pre-logical mentality which brought together fool, child and savage in a supposed proximity to the point of origin.

Chomsky's work programme, which saw syntax as an organ, opened the doors that this prohibition had slammed shut. If it is an organ, then it rightfully falls within the remit of evolutionary theory. Chomsky's refusal to this day to credit with any interest the contributions from the evolutionary perspective on language does reformulate, however, one of the pillars of the linguistic heritage. It is against this backdrop that we can read the importance of the recent paleontological dating that has been presented here by Bernard Victorri and Éric Saïer. They link the debate on the origin of mankind to the question of language. To this we must add the recent archaeological discoveries which in one fell swoop have pushed back by some 30,000 years the date for the first known fabrication of jewellery by African *homo sapiens* (Allemand, 2004, p. 47).[2] So too we must add the recent dynamic developments in human sciences such as the cognitive psychology that has been put together in correlation with the Chomskyan research programme and the evolutionary psychology that has been constructed as a derivation on bio-sociology. At a time when Chomskyism seems to be setting the pace, these disciplines are taking up the baton. This dynamism is undoubtedly a major factor behind the title and the originality of the conference that brings us together today.

Symbol-use as the sign of the origin of humankind has since Darwin set at least three camps at odds: those who side for a progressive refinement of the biological apparatus that enables humans to speak; those who side for its sudden genetic mutation; and the advocates of mixed solutions and more varied adjustments. For the moment, I won't be dealing with the place and role in this process of the distinction between Theory of Mind (ToM) and the capacity to speak as such; nor the distinction as to whether Theory of Mind is selected as a "meme" or whether it is the product of a module. Nor is it certain that psychoanalysis should have any need of the syntax organ as a condition for the unconscious. The materialism of the inscription of apparatuses of subjectivity is quite sufficient for this condition (Miller & Etchegoyen, 1996, p. 33).

In its Freudian tradition, psychoanalysis sided for sudden breakpoints. This is Freud's strange Lamarcko-Darwinism that reads the cause of a generalised anxiety in the glacial periods and the loss of the subject's environment. We will be coming back to this. Lacan took up this tradition by underlining the sudden cut-off point produced by the coupling between language and living being, a veritable trauma for the human species. He generalises Freudian castration by separating it from any notion of a threat voiced by an agent (the father of the horde or the *paterfamilias*) and reads human sexuality as a post-traumatic reconstruction. If we allow ourselves a slight exaggeration, we could say that human sexuation breaks with the animal unity of the species and produces two radically separate sub-species. With language, each of these two sub-species loses the definition of its partner and then has to go via the vast detour of language in order to retrieve the lost object and the remainder of jouissance that is reserved for it in the fantasmatic machinery. This is also a way of underlining the fact that jouissance, which implies a continuum between pleasure and what lies beyond the pleasure principle, cannot be reduced to incentive motivation in the limbic system.

Symptom, fantasy, and trauma were always linked for Freud, albeit in a distinct manner. At the outset, in 1895, Freud understood neurosis and the syndrome of traumatic repetition as being bound together. In his description of anxiety hysteria he mentions night waking followed by a syndrome of repetition and nightmares.[3] It was only after having isolated the death drive that he would separate recurrent dreams from hysteria, and would speak, with respect to the syndrome of traumatic repetition, of a failure of neurotic repetition, a failure of the defences, and a failure of the "protective shield against stimuli" (Freud, 1920g). In 1926, when he modifies the sense of "the trauma of birth" first identified by his pupil Otto Rank, Freud attributes the energetic conceptions that he had previously entertained to moments of anxiety in the face of essential loss. Freud distinguishes with great precision between birth and what arises from the traumatic loss of the maternal object properly speaking. He dares to read the necessary loss of the mother as the model for all other traumas.[4] It is against this backdrop that we should understand the aphorism from an almost contemporary text, the 1925 article "Negation", where the aim is "not to *find*" the object, but always "to *refind* such an object". It is always to be found against the backdrop of a primordial loss (Freud, 1925h).[5]

Lacan took the Freudian unconscious and the fundamental loss that is central to it and translated them using terms from the thought of the twentieth century, the same that was called the century of the "linguistic turn". In the course of the century, from different philosophical traditions, Frege, Russell, Husserl, and others, accentuated the drama that leads to the fact that once we are in language, we can no longer get out of it. This is what the first Wittgenstein stated in his pessimistic thesis that philosophy can only demonstrate tautologies and so the world can only "show" itself through other aesthetic, moral, and religious discourses. The breach in discourse is produced by *monstration*; the rest is tautology. To Wittgenstein's list we should add, with psychoanalysis, a breach by sex.

Lacan rewords Freud's thesis thus: we come into the world with a parasite known as the unconscious. Our "species-specific" trait is the combination of language with the bungling of sexual satisfaction. Psychoanalysis reckons not only on syntax but also on the bungling of sex. Our representations have a hole in them, that of the partner of whom we nevertheless continually dream, whom we continually hallucinate and strive to meet through the experience of jouissance. We can form for ourselves as many meta-representations as we wish: the sexual partner as such will still bear the stamp of an impossible. In his recent book *In Gods We Trust*, Scott Atran speaks of the "evolutionary landscape of religion" (Atran, 2002).[6] He deduces the gods from the very possibility that meta-representations offer of stretching the domain of a module beyond its effective domain. Since he hypothesises a module that recognises and classifies living beings, this module can then apply itself to meta-representations of non-living beings that are treated as living beings, as veritable supernatural creatures. Belief in the sexual partner is something of the same order: a meta-representation starting off from the "jouissance module" that is centred on the *refound* object (in the Freudian sense). At the very moment we learn to speak, we experience something that lives in a different way from the living being, and this is language and its significations, which fairly quickly take on an autonomous existence for the subject, as "false belief reasoning" in cognitive psychology bears out. Freud gave a significant place to the *proton pseudos*, the "original lie" (Freud, 1895a, p. 356), and Melanie Klein gave a similar place to the power of the "no" in constructing the subject's world. In the same move by which we communicate our libidinal demand and exigency, we discover the limits of this communication. We experience language as a wall. If we are not overly crushed by the misunderstanding in our exchanges with those we love, we nonetheless manage to speak. And so we come to experience the fact that we will only ever leave language by means of some breach or ecstatic transport.

On the fringes of the language system, a certain number of clinical phenomena are produced which fall within the category of the real, a real that is specific to the speaking being. These phenomena stand at once on the edge of this system and at its heart. They stem from a topology that is more complex than a mere inside and outside. Trauma, hallucination, and the experience of "perverse" jouissance all belong to this category. Neurotics too experience moments of anxiety that give them some idea of these phenomena and pull them away from their tendency to consider life as a dream.

As a way of taking this into account, Lacan proposes as of 1953 to inscribe language within a particular enclosed space, the torus, "in so far as the peripheral exteriority and central exteriority of a torus constitute but one single region" (Lacan, 2006, p. 264).

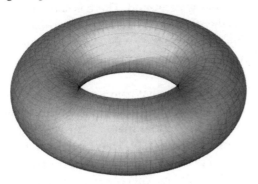

This model has the particularity of designating an interior that is also an exterior. It is profoundly linked to the conception of space in general. Reflections on topology allow us to move towards "progressive liberation from the notion of distance in geometry" (Luminet, 2008, p. 262)[7] and also from psychical "distance" with respect to a trauma.

The torus is the most straightforward form of space that includes a hole. So, in a first sense, trauma is a hole that lies within the symbolic. Here, the symbolic is posited as the system of the *Vorstellungen* through which the subject aims to refind the presence of a lost object. Here, the symbolic includes both the symptom in its formal envelope and also that which does not manage to be absorbed into it, the real point that remains exterior to any symbolic representation, whether symptom or unconscious fantasy. This allows the real to be figured in an "exclusion that is internal to the symbolic". "The symptom can appear as a repetitive statement about the real. [...] [It] is the subject's response to the traumatic aspect of the real" (Miller, 1998, p. 63). Here I am reproducing the diagram proposed by Jacques-Alain Miller which represents this real point:

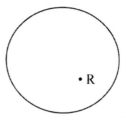

The Symbolic

The relationships between subject and symbolic may also be approached the other way around. There is something of the symbolic in the real: this is the *structure* of language, the existence of the language in which the child is caught, the pool of language into which he falls. In this sense, language conforms to the Theory-of-Mind supposition of speech functions.

We do not learn the rules that compose the Other of the social bond for us. Language as real is a tongue that escapes the system of language rules, a system that is no more than a "harebrained lucubration", as Lacan puts it (Lacan, 1998a, p. 139). The meaning of the rules is invented in starting off from a primordial point that lies outside meaning, a point of "attachment" to the Other. This is a perspective that is closer to late Wittgenstein and his argument on the constitution of a "community of life" that forms a primordial pragmatics. From this angle, after the trauma of loss, one has to reinvent an Other that no longer exists. Thus "caused", the subject now re-finds the rules of life with an Other that has been lost. In Freudian terms, one invents one's symptom and one's fantasy by overcoming the anxiety of the loss of the mother, the anxiety "caused" by the mother. One does not "learn" to live with the lost Other, and there is no pedagogy of reconciliation with life. One has to invent one's own "private language" from the contingency of events that surrounded the loss, from the public language shared with the Other one addresses. The status of language in the real may be noted as follows:

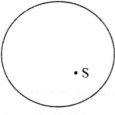

The Real

In yet another way, the immersion in language is traumatic because at its centre it bears a non-relation. The goal that is targeted—re-finding the lost partner—is never achieved. This is what Lacan calls *le non-rapport sexuel*, sexual non-relation. This non-relation is the experience of the variety of symptoms and fantasies that vouch for the fact that there is also a missing rule that has to be invented, yet which is forever wanting. In both cases, this inscription of the relationships between the real and the symbolic breaks with any relationship of modelling the real through the symbolic, which would merely be a reflection of the real in a relationship of exteriority.

It is on the basis of this experience, the subject's experience of his origin in the experience of loss that structures human jouissance, that I would like to read the different contributions to today's conference from its various participants, by indicating how they have helped me to gain a better grasp of the paradoxes and oddities of this jouissance.

Cognition and emotion

I shall start with the contributions from Pierre Jacob who broadly examines the relationships between stimulus and action on the basis of the Theory-of-Mind notion of a general capacity of attribution. I find the distinctions that he has set out and developed between motor representations and visual representations to be decisive. He thereby sets limits to the temptation "to use the concept of mental simulation as a theoretical basis to unify motor cognition and social cognition" (Jacob, 2004). These reservations have been abundantly useful for me. I recently heard a paper by a colleague from University College London, who also has links with the Tavistock Clinic through his psychoanalytic interests, in which he managed to reconstruct social cognition in its entirety on the basis of the organ for the Imaginary that is endued by "mirror neurone systems" (Rizzolatti et al., 2001). Furthermore, evolutionary psychology allowed him to argue out a basis for the evolutionary utility of aggressiveness in the reinforcement of "in-group" identifications, and then to demonstrate how the constraints of civilisation take over in order to obtain the same utility. From this he concluded that, as we continue down our evolutionary path, we should soon be able to abandon the archaic aspects of aggressiveness so as to pursue the same ends of group reinforcement through social rules properly speaking. In sum, we would purportedly be getting to what Robert Kagan called, when referring to the gap between the American and European positions, a veritable reconciliation between Hobbes and Kant, or between Mars and Venus (Kagan, 2002).

In his rejection of the Freudian death drive, which was so disturbing by virtue of the fault-line that it introduced with respect to the reduction of the subject to biological mechanisms, this author was pursuing a Kleinian current in which a number of excellent authors have distinguished themselves. Take for example Roger Money-Kyrle who in 1955 wrote:

> [B]efore accepting the death instinct, that is, the existence of an instinct with a self-destructive aim which cannot have been evolved by selection to promote survival, we must do our best to see how far the analytic facts can be explained without it. (Money-Kyrle, 2001, p. 503)

So, I am interested in these fine distinctions that Pierre Jacob has set out, but I would also like to turn to a very widespread effect on psychoanalysis that is generated by these too hasty borrowings from advances in neuroscience. These borrowings can produce conservative effects and freeze up specifically psychoanalytic debates, which are falsely resolved by this kind of borrowing. We can see this in authors like Mark Solms when he believes he has found Freud's second topography inscribed in the brain, or in the uncritical borrowing of the notion of "mental image" that some neuroscientists have gladly been employing without it being indispensable to their enterprise.

When Dan Sperber presents the seminal theses of Paul Grice, he carefully stresses that the latter's approach does not presuppose any hypotheses that may be equated with the "mental image" hypothesis:

According to the inferential model, different versions of which have been developed in contemporary pragmatics, an utterance is a piece of evidence of the speaker's meaning. Decoding the linguistic sentence meaning is seen as just one part of the process of comprehension—a process that relies on both this linguistic meaning and on the context in order to identify the speaker's meaning. [...] Meaning, in Grice's analysis, [...] is an intention to achieve a certain effect upon the mind of the hearer by means of the hearer's recognition of the very intention to achieve this effect.

Seen this way, communication depends upon the ability of human beings to attribute mental states to others; that is, it depends upon their naïve psychology [...]. Living in a world inhabited not only by physical objects and living bodies, but also by mental states, humans may want to act upon these mental states. They may seek to change the desires and beliefs of others. (Orrigi & Sperber, 2004)[8]

This presentation covers elements of what Pierre Jacob has presented to us. According to Grice, in the subject's activity, the Other is reached by going via a prior questioning as to the other party's intention. Therefore, there can be no production of meaning without a willingness to decipher intention. Lacan's formula that the subject receives from the Other his own message in an inverted form includes this *intention-to-be-deciphered*, but also integrates a critique of the code/message model. Indeed, it is ultimately a matter of reaching in the Other the partner of the fantasy.

It is by no means certain that the different currents of cognitivism have carried this initial Grice-inspired programme through to its end as a research programme. Take for example the programme of emotional cognitivism, which replaces the *processes of inference* with *processes of perception* by maintaining that a feeling is the cognitive perception of an emotion. Antonio Damasio is the paradigmatic author of this approach.

In their monumental *Philosophical Foundations of Neuroscience* which recently appeared, Bennett and Hacker present his position critically:

Antonio Damasio's work on patients suffering from emotionally incapacitating brain damage is rightly renowned, and his insistence on a link between the capacity for rational decision-making and consequent rational action in pursuit of goals, on the one hand, and the capacity for feeling emotions, on the other, is bold and thought-provoking. However, his speculations on the emotions are, in our view, vitiated by conceptual confusion. [...] Damasio's conception of thoughts is firmly rooted in the eighteenth-century empiricist tradition. Thoughts, he claims, consist of mental images (which may be visual or auditory etc ..., and may be of items in the world or of words or symbols that signify such items). Damasio apparently holds the view that if thought were not exhibited to us in the form of images of things and images of words signifying things, then we would not be able to say what we think. [...] Damasio distinguishes an emotion from the feeling of an emotion. An emotion is a bodily response to a mental image, and the feeling of an emotion is a cognitive response to that bodily condition, a cognitive response "in connection to the object that excited it, the realisation of the nexus between object and emotional body state". Feelings of emotion, Damasio avers, are just as cognitive as any other perceptual image, and just as dependent on cerebral-cortex processing as any other image. (Bennett & Hacker, 2003, pp. 210–211)

So, the notion of "mental image" is essential to Damasio, and despite his critiques of Descartes he does not seem to have rid himself of presuppositions about representation such as it was conceived of in the seventeenth century.

Ian Hacking takes issue with Damasio's version of his theory as outlined in the latter's most recent book, *Looking For Spinoza: Joy, Sorrow, and the Feeling Brain*:

[According to Damasio] "Emotions play out in the theatre of the body. Feelings in the theatre of the mind." Both are *for* "life regulation" but feelings do it at a higher level. Joy is the feeling of a life in equilibrium, sorrow of life in disarray ("functional disequilibrium"). [...]

Both feelings and emotions are states, conditions, or processes in the body. An emotion such as pity "is a complex collection of chemical and neural responses forming a distinctive pattern." Moreover, for Damasio there is nothing [...] "outer-directed". [...] For him pity is not of or about someone. And emotions seem to be caused by changes in [one's] body. [...]

> [This is] an inadequate theory, for you cannot have emotions without cognitive input [...]—that is perhaps the majority opinion of neurologists. (Hacking, 2004a, pp. 32–33)

Damasio's conception is of an Otherless organism, a profoundly autistic organism focused on its homeostatic auto-regulation and progressively refined throughout the course of evolution. Hacking says that:

> What he chooses to call emotions come first, historically speaking, in the history of evolution, and they are first causally, as the items that instigate a cycle of responses within the body. They produce feelings in another part of the brain, one that evolved later, and are in turn monitored and used in what he calls mind. (Hacking, 2004a, p. 33)

The meaning of the vocabulary of affects is thus ultimately none other than the precise emotion that is felt in the body. Damasio holds that it is possible to perform a one-to-one mapping of *feelings* onto bodily states (*emotions*). No more metaphorical or metonymical sliding would be possible, despite the fact that the register of affects is part and parcel of language. This is what Hacking is criticising:

> Feelings and emotions have been part of the language of persons, both for expressing my self and for describing others. Damasio proposes something different: instant anatomical identification of emotions; this is what they really are, that is what joy is. [...]
>
> [...] [T]here seems in Damasio's account to be no "I" left who decides how to handle [any given] situation. There is just self-regulating homeostasis going on in this organism. [...]
>
> Damasio will surely go on lobbying for an identification of the personal language with current anatomical conjectures. (Hacking, 2004a, pp. 35–36)

I fear that a number of psychoanalysts, including one author who is well known to Marc Jeannerod, the director of the institute that is hosting us so comfortably today—I'm referring to the current president of the International Psycho-Analytic Association—give a description of psychoanalytic activity that makes uncritical use of notions of "mental representation" such as Damasio employs. Thus, Daniel

Widlöcher writes that, "the analyst's listening is occupied with mental representations constructed by references taken from the analysand's words" (Widlöcher, 1996, p. 135). This is how he sets forth his "communicational" conception of the unconscious, the first condition of which is the capacity to attribute to the other party a Theory of Mind.

> The Theory of Mind in question stems from what the cognitivists call the capacity to *mind-read*. For an interpretation to be heard by the patient, a certain number of conditions are necessary. The first condition is that both interlocutors share a certain Theory of Mind. (Widlöcher, 1996, p. 135)

Theory of mind strikes him as being a prerequisite for the mode of inference that leads to interpretation. Thus he terms "empathy" the inference that gives him access to the meaning of what the analysand says, "meaning that lies beyond a mere decoding of the signified" (Widlöcher, 1996, p. 143). This research into mental state comes at a price:

> At the end of the day, the words are always missing in psychoanalytic communication. For want of precise and reciprocal conversational imperatives, mental states take on a chaotic and fluctuating character that forbids any clear idea from being extracted from them. [...] Analytic comprehension affords a view of a labour of inference that knows no end. [...] If we push the paradox further, we could say that the ideal session would be this dual silence. (Widlöcher, 1996, p. 147)

Can one really say that an "ideal" session would be one in which both parties would at last fall silent, each having withdrawn into the jouissance of their auto-erotic inference? Grice's inference emerges from this utterly transformed into a limitless process. This is an odd way to encounter the limitlessness of language.

Bernard Victorri's narrative and the Freudian Witz

Bernard Victorri's text struck me as especially interesting to the extent that the functionalist approach that he develops mirrors the psychoanalytic subversion of the code/message linguistic model so as to raise the question of the origin of novelty in natural languages. This dynamics of novelty caught my attention, as did his accentuation of "dynamic situations" described in natural languages, and, more generally, his choice to broach syntax via semantics.

The approach to modalities and deictics that he puts forth from this perspective imparts to the subject's relations with the world a description that does not make do with a simple inside/outside opposition. Describing modal verbs in terms of *access* does not create any other exterior besides the very process of narration itself. In this way it produces a functionalist speech space, which is reminiscent of the "function of speech" that Lacan isolated in "Function and field of speech and language in psychoanalysis" (Lacan, 2006, pp. 197–268). Let's look first at how the modalities immerse us into this space:

> The access from the previous scenes to the new one can be necessary (no other path towards another situation), just possible (at least two paths leading one to the evoked new scene and the other not), or impossible (no path to the new scene). These distinctions are the most important ones from the point of view of a narrative process in which each new scene is constructed from what is already present in the intersubjective space produced by previous discourse. (Victorri, 2007, p. 3)

When it comes to deictics, the functional choice that Victorri makes goes in the same direction:

> If we accept the idea that the main objective of language is to give a phenomenological presence to all the entities and events evoked by discourse, it is obvious that the use of the same markers for referring to real as well as discourse entities is a very efficient way to endow these discourse entities with the same unquestionable presence in the intersubjective space. In fact, language appears as a better device to give strength to the phenomenological existence of what is said, than to secure transmission of factual information. (Victorri, 2007, p. 4)[9]

The approach to syntax then follows on from the same perspective:

> [A]nother important set of syntactic phenomena, which has been emphasised by functional grammar theorists [...] concerns all

the syntactic mechanisms offered by languages to introduce new entities, events and relations (which are called "new information" or "focus" or "rheme"), by "anchoring" them into a framework composed by the entities, events and relations already shared with the addressee [...]. It is clear that these mechanisms are of particular interest for narrative purposes, since the success of a narration depends crucially on the capacity of evoking new characters or events on the unique basis of what has already been put on the stage. (Victorri, 2007, p. 4)

Another of Victorri's perspectives also caught my attention: his presentation of the dead ends of *hominisation* and the distance he takes from a linear vision of development. He gives a very interesting version of man as an "evolution-sick animal".

In humankind [...] social regulation does not happen at the biological level, but at the socio-cultural level. [...] [T]his means that in humans the biological control of behaviours that present a danger for the species are inexistent or at the very least considerably weakened. [...] In other words, the development of individual intelligence had its corollary in the loss of instinctive reactions, including, ultimately, those reactions which were most firmly established because they were vital to the survival of the species, such as those that regulate aggressiveness within groups.[10]

Victorri's formulation of the woes of cognition leads us to the appointment with the suffering of thought:

This same evolutionary pressure led to an almost total domination of the neocortex that endangered the species by weakening the instinctive constraints that formerly regulated social life. [...] It is simply a matter of giving a concrete illustration of a general principle: the development of individual intelligence can generate antisocial behaviour that is harmful to the survival of the species. In the absence of biological or social constraints that would be able to stem its effects, the *Homo* branch found itself submitted for an entire period to social crises that can explain the inherent weakness that we have qualified as an evolutionary dead end.[11]

This presents us with a schema that profoundly complicates the simplicity of a mechanical reading of Freud's second topography, with an *id* that drives, a *superego* that inhibits, and an *ego* that survives by virtue of its "Perception-Consciousness System".

Freud had supposed that the legislating father was a relic of the privations that arose in the last glacial period:

> Our first hypothesis would thus maintain that mankind, under the influence of the privations that the encroaching Ice Age imposed upon it, has become generally *anxious*. The hitherto predominantly friendly outside world, which bestowed every satisfaction, transformed itself into a mass of threatening perils. There had been good reason for realistic anxiety about everything new. [...] As the hard times progressed, the primal humans, whose existence was threatened, must have been subjected to the conflict between self-preservation and the desire to procreate [...] The subsequent evolution is easy to construct. It primarily affected the male. After he had learned to economise on his libido and by means of regression to degrade his sexual activity to an earlier phase, activating his intelligence became paramount for him. [...] It is the time of the animistic worldview and its magical trappings. As a reward for his power to safeguard the lives of so many other helpless ones he bestowed upon himself unrestrained dominance over them, and through his personality established the first two tenets that he was himself invulnerable and that his possession of women must not be challenged. At the end of this epoch the human race had disintegrated into individual hordes that were dominated by a strong and wise brutal man as father. (Freud, 1987, pp. 13–16)

Bernard Victorri also reads social invention as a competitive advantage, but he places the invention of narrative poetics prior to the invention of law:

> [E]ven if it happened rarely, a successful outcome [of such a "narrative trick"] would have had immediate consequences for the survival of the group in which it took place. Therefore, it could have generalised in the long run, exactly like an advantageous genetic trait, which spreads over a species by natural selection rules. One

important step in this process could have been the "ritualisation" of the narrative behaviour: instead of waiting for the outbreak of a crisis, it would have been much more efficient to organise regular events in which the famous ancestors and the prohibited acts were evoked. (Victorri, 2007, p. 8)

A "narrative function" employed by the new legislators enables "our species to control the social disturbances that could explain the extinction of the other archaic *Homo sapiens*" (Victorri, 2007, p. 8).

It seems to me that it is perfectly possible to subscribe to Victorri's final thesis of the *Homo narrans*:

> It is in this spirit that we have presented this thesis, which sees man as a *Homo narrans* because it is not intelligence that would distinguish him from the other species of *Homo sapiens* that came before him, but the capacity to tell his own story, the wellspring of a new founding "wisdom" for human societies.[12]

To my mind, this presentation of *Homo narrans* joins up with the function that Lacan attributes to the Freudian *Witz* in his fifth Seminar (Lacan, 1998b). The *Witz* is above all a new signifier that escapes the code. From this perspective, only those signifiers that escape the code really "make sense". They must, however, come to be inscribed in the "family" of signifiers that already exist. This is why, in his remarkable commentary on this Seminar, Jacques-Alain Miller notes:

> The *Witz* is first and foremost this: something new in the fact of saying. The principial example that he sets off from, which since then has resonated for us, is Henrich Heine's "famillionairely". It is a word that had never been uttered, a creation, a novelty. [...] The witticism is only really accomplished once the Other has recognised it as such. This difference is then sanctioned by the Other as a flash of wit. (Miller, 2000, pp. 12–15)

He continues: "The crux of it lies in not disconcerting the Other. You still have to obtain his acquiescence, his consent. You still need him to say 'yes'" (Miller, 2000, p. 19). This acquiescence at one remove presupposes a public language that is recognised as such by a group: a social bond in Lacan's sense of the term.

> There is no flash of wit in abstract space. This is congruent with what Lacan set out thereafter: the one thing that he salvages from Bergson's book on *Laughter*, namely, that the other party has to be from the same parish. For there to be a witticism, the other party has to understand you, and for that, he has to be from the same vicinity. The parish is a limited Other. It's neither the universe nor a list of dignitaries, nor is it the whole of Christendom. The parish is a neighbourhood. [...] It's like with a baby's babbling: if it isn't put up with and welcomed in a certain way, it perishes. First of all it has to be put up with, the Other has to smile at it, and so on. Even our neuroscientist colleagues have confirmed that it takes an other party who smiles before the neurones start functioning as they should. (Miller, 2000, pp. 26–32)

Moreover, what interests us in this Seminar is that Lacan generates the father function, the Name-of-the-Father, from its function in the poetics of the *Witz*:

> In this Seminar, the Name-of-the-Father is definitively that which in the code can say "yes" to neologisms. [...] The Name-of-the-Father is this function which represents the Law so as to be able at the same time to welcome the exception. (Miller, 2000, pp. 36–37)

The father according to Lacan cannot be reduced to the father who forbids or the father of the primal scene. This father is the one who favours the emergence of a new signifier.

You can understand, therefore, that Bernard Victorri's perspective has held my attention just as Scott Atran's has, as we are about to see. This function of welcoming what is new is certainly crucial for our civilisation to be able to cope with the growing impasses that its programme is meeting, rather than trusting blindly in the evolutionary inheritance given us at the outset.

The Darwinism of jouissance and cultural nominalism

Scott Atran presents a version of the "cognitive theory of culture" conceived of as a radical cultural nominalism: "culture *per se*" is not a well-defined entity (neither a system of rules, mores, or norms, nor a code or a grammar of symbols or behaviours) nor is it a "super organism".

It is a fluid distribution of private and public representations, natural and artificial ecological conditions that channel and relay represented information (seas, mountains, edifices, paper, etc.) and the behaviours that arise from them. This distributive conception of culture stands in opposition to a conception based on the usual social science and cognitive notions of culture, such as a) the error of conceiving of culture as a delimited system or an independent variable, and b) the tendency to "essentialise" culture and to treat it as an explanation and not as a phenomenon to be explained. Just as it was (and remains) hard for biology to reject the essentialist concept of "species" (as a well-defined entity with its own structure) in favour of "species" as an historic lineage of individuals, it is also hard to abandon the popular notion of culture as a body endued with its own essence (a system of rules, norms or practices) (Atran, 2004).[13]

I would like to situate Atran's perspective as that of a radical nominalist, and relate it to the biological conceptions developed by Pierre Sonigo and Jean-Jacques Kupiec. In his section of the book that he authored with Sonigo, *Ni Dieu ni gène*, Kupiec sets Darwin into a wider English filiation, making him a radical heir to William of Ockham's nominalism:

> Repeating in biology what Ockham had done five centuries earlier for metaphysics, Darwin abandons the ideal entities that haunted his precursors to turn instead to real individuals. This definition no longer translates an immutable property of the species, such as the possession of a characteristic structure (specific difference) or the fact of not being able to mix with members of another species, but the mechanism of evolution itself, i.e. the variation that lies at its base. Darwin's definition does not say what species are, but what they do. The species is not a static entity. What is involved is a process. With this abandonment of specificity, Darwin opened the possibility of a new biological theory that broke away from Aristotle's metaphysics. (Kupiec & Sonigo, 2000, p. 49)

The criticism that he gives of a genetic ideology as the realisation of a programme that is already written out interests us because it offers a critique of the more comprehensive notion of language reduced to a code/message mechanism. From the perspective of the programme, a continuous chain establishes a mechanism in which the programme contains the essence of the living being in a discrete form that can be duly decoded. The genome is thus thought of as a veritable divine writing of the living being. Kupiec and Sonigo call this into question, thereby justifying the title of their book, a book that goes so far as to cast doubt on the necessity of a "programme" and its determinism.

> From the 'sixties and 'seventies on, the genomes of pluricellular organisms were analysed in ever greater detail, which allowed for some unexpected characteristics to be brought to light that are still hard to explain within the framework of deterministic models: redundancy, non-coding DNA, recombinations and point mutations. (Kupiec & Sonigo, 2000, pp. 112–113)

The contingency of a topological position and selection by a host environment could be more important for the activation of a gene than its signification as determined by a so-called programme.

For us, this perspective echoes the texts we have examined and also the situation that Lacan describes of a *symbolic in the real*. Lacan determines a space in which the signifier is no longer the master that reiterates a rule. The signifier passes over to the function of an instrument of jouissance as a means of expression for the fantasy. The Other as a system is articulated with equivocal "odds and ends of the real" that constantly give rise to multiple readings. *Equivocation* stands in the foreground of this conception, forming an obstacle to any essentialist representation of reading and writing. In a world of partial readings, the topology of the signifier enables the equivocal twisting of chains that are ever more supple, folding to the constraints of a jouissance which does not seek to be spoken, but which makes use of the symbolic in order to enjoy *encore*.

Far from a rigid and frozen definition of the law of language or of the mechanics of the second topography, the contributions from Pierre Jacob, Bernard Victorri and Scott Atran have allowed me to form a grasp of this bond with the Other that is articulated on the basis of elements and fragments, without for all that having to take on board any notion of representation or of mental images, both of which inevitably refer back to a preceding whole.

Psychoanalysis, which is not a naturalist psychology, is able to take into account the displacements of its problematic by the discoveries of science. It is also able to warn us against one of the illusions of evolutionary psychology: the excess of belief in an order of Nature that would absorb the aporias that lie between the Other, civilisation, and jouissance.

At a time when Nature no longer exists, when she has been replaced by "the environment", and at a time when science can no longer provide us with "the theory of everything", the danger that an overly strong belief in the just-so stories of evolutionary psychology presents is to end up with a return to good old Nature and her orderly state. This *Aufhebung* would soon reveal itself as the fairytale for the children of science that it is. It would be a way of restoring belief in Father Christmas, of which psychoanalysis was designed to rid us.

Notes

1. See Dr Saïer's "Allocution d'accueil" to the conference *Origine de l'homme et souffrance psychique*, at the Institut des Sciences Cognitives, Lyon, 6 November 2004.
2. "There are thirty-nine of these beads fashioned from shells. [...] Made some 75, 000 years ago, their discovery pushes back by thirty thousand years the date when bodies were first adorned with jewellery, and with it the date for the first fabrication of symbolic objects. What's more, they were found deep in the Southern African continent, when previously the oldest known pendants came from Bulgaria and Turkey." (Allemand, 2004, p. 47).
3. The *pavor nocturnus* of adults that Freud outlines in point 5 of Freud, 1895b.
4. Addendum C to Freud, 1926d, p. 171: "In consequence of the infant's misunderstanding of the facts, the situation of missing its mother is not a danger-situation but a traumatic one. [...] Thus, the first determinant of anxiety, which the ego itself introduces, is loss of perception of the object (which is equated with loss of the object itself). [...] The traumatic situation of missing the mother differs in one important respect from the traumatic situation of birth. At birth no object existed and so no object could be missed."
5. The original German reads: "Der erste und nächste Zweck der Realitätsprüfung ist also nicht, ein dem Vorgestellten entsprechendes Objekt in der realen Wahrnehmung zu finden, sondern es wiederzufinden, sich zu überzeugen, daß es noch vorhanden ist." ("Die Verneinung" in *Gesammelte Werke*, vol. XIV, Fischer Verlag, 1948, p. 14).

6. See too the review: Hacking, 2004b. [Scott Atran participated in the *Origine de l'homme et souffrance psychique* conference with the paper "Origine et évolution de la culture humaine".]

7. This is determined on the basis of a magnitude that was defined by Simon Lhuilier in 1813 as the *genus* of any given closed surface: "It can also be defined for any type of closed surface, and it is then called the *genus*. The genus of the torus is 1, that of a sphere is 0, and that of a sphere equipped with H handles is H." (Luminet, 2008, p. 262).

8. [What is translated here as "naïve psychology" might also be rendered as "Theory of Mind" (Tr.).]

9. [The original French text (published in *Langages*, Vol. 36, Issue 146, 2002, pp. 112–125) has *simulation de perception* where the English has "the phenomenological existence of what is said" (Tr.)]

10. [Our translation of the 2002 French version in view of the considerably re-written 2007 English version. The reader may wish to compare the passage reproduced here with section III from the 2007 text: "The problem of the near total extinction of archaic *Homo sapiens*", pp. 5–7. (Tr.)]

11. [As per preceding note (Tr.).]

12. [As per preceding note (Tr.).]

13. See also: Atran, 2003.

CHAPTER SIX

The cul-de-sac of cognitive psychoanalysis

The following paper was published in La Cause freudienne, *issue 60, June 2005, pp. 17–22.**

Cognitive psychoanalysis, and neuropsychoanalysis with it, bear witness to the impact that the neurosciences have had on our discipline and the manner in which the latter have taken it on board. We must, therefore, distinguish between the results of the neurosciences properly speaking and the ways in which they are integrated into the different psychoanalytic orientations. An examination of this reception, a mode of reception which can go so far as the "abusive importing of concepts" from the neurosciences (as Louis Althusser might have put it), is all the more important given how the interface between psychoanalysis and the neurosciences has been steadily extending its reach.

---

* An earlier version of this article was translated into English by Lieve Billiet as "The Blind Alleys of Cognitive Psychoanalysis" in the *Lacanian Review of Psychoanalysis*, Issue 2.

Coincidences

The March 2004 IPA Congress, held in New Orleans, was marked by the momentous invitation of professor Antonio Damasio, a neuroscientist known for his sympathies for psychoanalysis. As Daniel Widlöcher reported in the 23 August 2004 edition of *L'Express*: "The auditorium was full, and he received a standing ovation. In other words, assimilating the thought of the likes of Damasio with the thought of a shrink poses no problems." (Widlöcher, 2004)

The most recent IPA Congress, on the theme of trauma, took place in Brazil in July 2005.[1] A large portion of it was given over to the cognitive approach and to the contributions to psychoanalysis from the neurosciences. Those present were also able to attend the Sixth International Congress of Neuro-Psychoanalysis, held at the same time, on the theme of "Dreams and Psychosis".

The Lacanian movement has seen similar *rapprochements*. One author has just published a book that aims to show how psychoanalysis can be perfectly compatible with the neurosciences (Pommier, 2004).

The various aspects of this tacit agreement ought to spell good news. Psychoanalysis would, indeed, thereby be confirmed in its scientific status by the simple fact that it is possible to translate its concepts and its experience into terms that have come from the neurosciences. Affirming this possibility brings consequences for psychoanalysis itself.

We are going to examine, therefore, the effects of this turn to emotional cognitivism as a way of accounting for affect in the analytic experience. This turn testifies to a push to establish a current of cognitivist psychoanalysis that would complement the contemporary version of ego psychology.

Antonio Damasio and the mental image of emotion

We have observed in particular the conservative effect of the impact of the neurosciences, an effect that is linked to an uncritical employment of the notion of "mental image".

This notion is not, however, indispensable to contemporary cognitivism, which has noble origins. We are referring here to a linguistic pragmatics that freed itself of the code/message model so as to focus on a process of a deductive inference. The name of the philosopher of language Paul Grice is particularly associated with this project. Gloria Origgi and Dan Sperber have presented this link as follows:

According to the inferential model, different versions of which have been developed in contemporary pragmatics, an utterance is a piece of evidence of the speaker's meaning. Decoding the linguistic sentence meaning is seen as just one part of the process of comprehension—a process that relies on both this linguistic meaning and on the context in order to identify the speaker's meaning. [...] Meaning, in Grice's analysis, [...] is an intention to achieve a certain effect upon the mind of the hearer by means of the hearer's recognition of the very intention to achieve this effect.

Seen this way, communication depends upon the ability of human beings to attribute mental states to others; that is, it depends upon their naïve psychology [...]. Living in a world inhabited not only by physical objects and living bodies, but also by mental states, humans may want to act upon these mental states. They may seek to change the desires and beliefs of others. (Orrigi & Sperber, 2004)[2]

Therefore, there can be no production of meaning without a willingness to decipher the other party's intention. Lacan's formula that the subject receives from the Other his own message in an inverted form includes this *intention-to-be-deciphered* and integrates a critique of the code/message model.

Now, it is by no means certain that any of the different currents of cognitivism have carried this research programme initiated by linguistic pragmatics through to its end. Take for example the programme of emotional cognitivism, which replaces the *processes of inference* with *processes of perception* by maintaining that a *feeling* is the cognitive perception of an *emotion*. Damasio is the paradigmatic author of this approach. In their monumental *Philosophical Foundations of Neuroscience* which recently appeared, Max Bennett and Peter Hacker present his position critically:

Antonio Damasio's work on patients suffering from emotionally incapacitating brain damage is rightly renowned, and his insistence on a link between the capacity for rational decision-making and consequent rational action in pursuit of goals, on the one hand, and the capacity for feeling emotions, on the other, is bold and thought-provoking. However, his speculations on the emotions are, in our view, vitiated by conceptual confusion. [...] Damasio's conception of thoughts is firmly rooted in the eighteenth-century empiricist tradition. Thoughts, he claims, consist of mental images (which may be visual or auditory etc ..., and may be of items in the world or of words or symbols that signify such items). Damasio apparently holds the view that if thought were not exhibited to us in the form of images of things and images of words signifying things, then we would not be able to say what we think. [...] Damasio distinguishes an emotion from the feeling of an emotion. An emotion is a bodily response to a mental image, and the feeling of an emotion is a cognitive response to that bodily condition, a cognitive response "in connection to the object that excited it, the realisation of the nexus between object and emotional body state". Feelings of emotion, Damasio avers, are just as cognitive as any other perceptual image, and just as dependent on cerebral-cortex processing as any other image. (Bennett & Hacker, 2003, pp. 210–211)

So, the notion of "mental image" is essential to Damasio, and despite his critiques of Descartes he does not seem to have rid himself of presuppositions about representation such as it was conceived of in the seventeenth century.

Ian Hacking takes issue with Damasio's version of his theory as outlined in the latter's most recent book, *Looking For Spinoza: Joy, Sorrow, and the Feeling Brain*:

[According to Damasio] "Emotions play out in the theatre of the body. Feelings in the theatre of the mind." Both are *for* "life regulation" but feelings do it at a higher level. Joy is the feeling of a life in equilibrium, sorrow of life in disarray ("functional disequilibrium"). [...]

Both feelings and emotions are states, conditions, or processes in the body. An emotion such as pity "is a complex collection of chemical and neural responses forming a distinctive pattern." Moreover, for Damasio there is nothing [...] "outer-directed". [...] For him pity is not of or about someone. And emotions seem to be caused by changes in [one's] body. [...]

[This is] an inadequate theory, for you cannot have emotions without cognitive input [...]—that is perhaps the majority opinion of neurologists. (Hacking, 2004a, pp. 32–33)

Damasio's conception is of an Otherless organism, a profoundly autistic organism focussed on its homeostatic auto-regulation and which is progressively refined throughout the course of evolution. As Hacking underlines, Damasio uses the term "emotion" for what comes first, historically speaking, in the history of evolution, as well as what comes first causally (because emotions are "the items that instigate a cycle of responses within the body"). Emotions are purported to produce "feelings" in another part of the brain, one that evolved later, and these are regulated by what he calls "mind" (Hacking, 2004a, p. 33).

The meaning of the vocabulary of affects is thus ultimately none other than the precise emotion that is felt in the body. Damasio holds that it is possible to perform a one-to-one mapping of *feelings* onto bodily states (*emotions*). No more metaphorical or metonymical sliding would be possible, despite the fact that the register of affects is part and parcel of language.

This is what Hacking is criticising:

> Feelings and emotions have been part of the language of persons, both for expressing my self and for describing others. Damasio proposes something different: instant anatomical identification of emotions; this is what they really are, that is what joy is. [...]
>
> [...] [T]here seems in Damasio's account to be no "I" left who decides how to handle [any given] situation. There is just self-regulating homeostasis going on in this organism. [...]
>
> Damasio will surely go on lobbying for an identification of the personal language with current anatomical conjectures. (Hacking, 2004a, pp. 35–36)

Abolishing equivocation in favour of representation

A certain "modernist" current in the IPA, which has been dominant in the Association's latter-day spheres of management, has sought to draw inspiration from the cognitive sciences in a twofold fashion. First, they took up the critique of the code/message approach so as to lean on the distinction between the language faculty and the Theory of Mind that all subjects attribute to others. Then, from emotional cognitivism, they took the inroad to an unequivocal definition of affect.

Peter Fonagy and Mark Solms[3] have offered a description of psychoanalytic activity by making uncritical use of the notion of "mental representation" employed by cognitivists. For both Fonagy and Solms, the analyst's listening is occupied with mental representations constructed by references taken from the analysand's words. This is how they have come to develop a "communicational" conception of the unconscious, the first condition of which is the capacity to attribute to the other party a Theory of Mind. The Theory of Mind in question stems from what cognitivists call the capacity to *mind-read*. As Widlöcher puts it:

> For an interpretation to be heard by the patient, a certain number of conditions are necessary. The first condition is that both interlocutors share a certain Theory of Mind. (Widlöcher, 1996, p. 135)

The Theory of Mind that is attributed to the other party establishes an imaginary version of the locus of the Other. According to these authors, it allows for the deployment of a particular mode of inference that would be specific to psychoanalysis. So it is that the recourse to "empathy" comes to define the possibility of accessing the meaning of what the analysand says, a meaning that purportedly lies beyond the decoding of the signified.

Let's compare this two-tier conception with Damasio's theory. For Damasio, there is first a "body state" perceived by the brain, which defines an emotion. Likewise, for the cognitivist psychoanalysts, the "body state" is transcribed into a "mental state" that corresponds to the "motive force of the drive". Next, there is an "effect of pleasure or displeasure" that takes into account the context in which this "motive force of the drive" comes to be set. The second phase can be superposed onto Damasio's "modelling", which sees "feeling" as something that is generated on the basis of the body-state perception constituted by "emotion".

Thus, this conception of affect as what sets the meaning of a subject's statement joins seamlessly with emotion as defined by Damasio's emotional cognitivism. All we have to do is replace Damasio's name in Hacking's review with that of a cognitive psychoanalyst to see a possible future for psychoanalysis as envisaged by the IPA: "They will surely go on lobbying for a reduction of personal language to current affective conjectures."

Cutting out the Other and reducing the body to an organism

The reformulation of psychoanalysis by means of the drafting-in of cognitive theories can take many different forms. One example is Fonagy in his co-authored book *Affect Regulation, Mentalization and the Development of the Self*. The confusional "false science" effect is guaranteed, regardless of the interest of the neurological research on which he draws. One critic who recently reviewed the book in the *Journal of the American Psychoanalytic Association* puts it unswervingly:

> [A]t times I found myself confused over the purpose of this work—since it is dealing primarily with cognitive processes and theory of mind, was it written for cognitive psychologists to demonstrate the ways in which psychoanalytic concepts can be located within their field? Or was the authors' intention to help analysts better appreciate ways in which psychoanalysis can be enriched by concepts such as learning theory, or by the fundamentals of biofeedback? [...] [A]t times the writing is dense and far from accessible; I found myself working hard to distil the ideas from the language they were couched in, and often wondered how they might be relevant to psychoanalysts. (Tyson, 2004, p. 631)

The standardising blind window of this version of cognition cuts out the Other. It presents us with a body reduced to an organism whose determination would condemn us to being no more than mere puppets of ourselves. Evolutionary psychology is playing the role of guarantor of this whole conception. It assures us that our organism and its psyche are perfectly functional because evolution so decrees. At a time when natural evidence is evaporating through the action of science, and at a time when science cannot guarantee any return to the order of a cosmos by means of a "theory of everything", evolutionism is peddling an *Aufhebung* of Nature. A reassuring natural order is being handed to us on a plate and evolutionary psychology is vouching for it. Emotion and cognition follow on one from the next, reinforcing each other as the order of evolution dictates. The programme of civilisation itself no longer knows any bounds. The irreducible dimension in the contradiction between drive and civilisation is vanishing. In this sense, turning to the neurosciences and to evolutionary psychology is on the one hand setting out an unfettered progressivism for civilisation and on the other orienting clinical treatment towards obtaining some form of joy for the self-regulated organism.

We have no need to draw on the neurosciences in such a way as to make out that they say the same thing as psychoanalysis or that they confirm it. Rather we should be distinguishing between the two planes of *scientific objectivity* and the *objectality of psychoanalysis*. The object *a* is not demonstrated by science. It is on the basis of the object *a* and the symptom[4] that we need to examine science's effect on the production of the subject and on the regime of its certainties. The principles of Lacanian psychoanalytic practice ground interpretation on the experience of a real that is specific to psychoanalysis, and not on any conformity with objects produced by a scientific discourse.

Notes

1. What a coincidence: the World Association of Psychoanalysis had held its Congress in Comandatuba in July 2004!
2. [What is translated here as "naïve psychology" might also be rendered as "Theory of Mind" (Tr.)]
3. Mark Solms, psychoanalyst and honorary lecturer in neurochemistry at St. Bartholomew's Hospital and the Royal London School of Medicine, is notably the author of *The Neuropsychology of Dreams: A Clinico-Anatomical Study* (Solms, 1997). See also Solms, 2004.
4. Here we are drawing on Jacques-Alain Miller's course from January 2005 (*L'orientation lacanienne III, 7, Pièces détachées*) in which he presents Lacan, 2005a.

CHAPTER SEVEN

Cognition and transference in psychoanalysis today

The following paper was presented at the Thirty-Third Study Days of the École de la Cause freudienne, Désangoisser avec la psychanalyse, held in Paris on 2–3 October 2004.

"Overcoming anxiety with psychoanalysis" may be read as the statement of a therapeutic project and the exploration of its limits. It may also be read as a willingness to place anxiety at the heart of the psychoanalytic process, to make it a touchstone for psychoanalysis. What place, what importance, and what treatment, does a psychoanalytic orientation give to anxiety? For us, anxiety is a reference point that does not deceive.

I would like, therefore, to examine in relation to this question two orientations that form two irreconcilable poles of psychoanalysis that lie beyond the confines of our orientation: on one hand, the cognitivist pole of the new ego psychology, and on the other, the practitioners of countertransference and the new object relations. We shall be looking at contemporary psychoanalysis as it goes in careful search of stable points by which it might ensure the certitude of its act. Next, we shall be seeing how this concern assumes an ordered frame on the basis of the touchstone of anxiety. We are also going to be meeting the foundations of a new symptom in the international psychoanalytic movement, which is placing the analytic cause in the hands of quantitative studies.

Leaving behind the entanglements of the imaginary

In an article that is crucial for our orientation, Jacques-Alain Miller has traced out the history and the current state of the notion of counter-transference in the IPA's theory of its practice. He pinpoints the mutation whereby a series of emotions has been brought to the fore at the expense of the singularity of anxiety:

> What already looks to be un-Freudian is the idea that the analyst's emotion is a response to the patient and that it is identical to the patient's most originary experiences, experiences which would then be legible on the side of the analyst. Indeed, this orientation utterly transforms the use of the Freudian experience because analysing the countertransference is thereafter likely to replace remembering and reconstructing the patient's past. Countertransference is supposed to give direct access to the patient's unconscious history—"direct" because the analyst *feels* it. (Miller, 2003b, translation modified)

This notion of the analyst's direct access to the analysand's history has given rise to some bizarre effects. Christopher Bollas, whose science-fiction article relating a catastrophic scenario was published in French translation in *La Cause freudienne*, describes what could happen to psychoanalysis:

> [F]or differing reasons and in varied ways analysands re-create their infantile life in the transference in such a determined and unconsciously accomplished way that the analyst is compelled to relive elements of this infantile history through his countertransference, his internal response to the analysand. (Bollas, 1987, p. 200)

Here it is being said, if we put it more mechanically, that the patient's psychical apparatus is being extended by the psychical apparatus of the analyst. More vampirically put: the analyst snatches hold of the psychical apparatus of the analysand. In a more mythical vein: the interaction between the two psychical apparatuses creates a "nowhere" locus that amounts to a "chimera". Lastly, in a more possessed style: "My words

[…] were uttered by my mouth, but they seemed to have been dictated from a place unknown to me, where the patient's associative discourse and my inner discourse interlink."[1]

Something along the lines of this "nowhere" locus has to exist for the analysts of one particular current in the IPA to consider that their interpretations do not come from themselves *qua* egos. Only an authorisation of this sort would purportedly allow for interpretation "in full flight" or, as one author has put it, "the interpretation whose advent precedes its very conception".

Effacing the dissymmetry between analyst and analysand also gives rise to unsettling effects with respect to the position of the analyst. It clouds the analyst's access to the knowledge that enables him to interpret and tie up the session with a quilting point. The practitioners that belong to this current are in search of the locus of insight that would give the analyst the certainty that, "all of a sudden, he knows". This support is indispensable when it comes to avoiding countertransferential acting-out. Insight belongs to the realm of knowledge that is obtained by the paths of the imaginary, as Jacques-Alain Miller has noted (Miller, 2003b).

These practitioners of countertransference are searching in different ways for the quilting point of the session. According to their own accounts, even our colleagues in the IPA are in search of a key experience such as this, with some of them drawing their interpretations from a "near-hallucinatory" state which they reach in the session and which removes them from the world of "normal" reasoning. Near-hallucination can also tip over onto the side of the analysand, furnishing the session with its quilting point. One author has written:

> Confronted with an abrupt rupture in the bindings of representations […] meaning emerges, for example, the regressive, sensory form, with anal characteristics, of a hallucinated smell. (Botella & Botella, 2005, p. 179)

We are not necessarily reassured by indications that these "hallucinatory" processes are specific modes of rational thought particular to the psychoanalyst. André Green speaks of "clinical thought" as one might say "savage thought";[2] and Michel de M'Uzan speaks of "paradoxical thought" as a way of situating this mode of understanding that is open to both the "paradoxes" of the unconscious and a maintained rationality. Under the label "clinical thought" they attempt to justify confused indications and an inadequate articulation between the imaginary, the symbolic and the real. This is precisely why Daniel Widlöcher's remarks reported in *L'Express* require some qualification:

> We consider that a frame set by the clock is needed to allow the patient to develop his thought associations, whilst for some, the Lacanians, one has to come to a key experience upon which the session is brought to a stop. (Widlöcher, 2004)

This quest for a key experience—one point, and that's it—does not necessarily lie on the side that he says it does.

Through this array of positions, and this quest for an anchoring of insight, we sense rather the difficulty these practitioners have in articulating transference in its guise of the repetition of the subject's fundamental signifiers and its centring around the object *a* that emerges in the chain of representations. To achieve such an articulation, there is really no need to stray off into talk about hallucinations.

To snatch from anxiety its certainty

To give an image of the structure of the transferential field, Lacan takes the metaphor of a hand reaching out to a log whereupon it bursts into flames and lights up the room. Before speaking about transference in *Seminar XI* as turning around the object *a* in the "enaction of the [sexual] reality of the unconscious" (Lacan, 1977b, p. 146), Lacan singled out the two sides of this field in *Seminar X*:

> I believe that the reference to transference, when limited solely to effects of reproduction and repetition, is too narrow and would deserve to be expanded. In insisting on the historical dimension, or on the repetition of lived experience, one runs the risk of sweeping aside a whole dimension that is no less important, the synchronic dimension, the dimension of what is precisely included, latent, in the position of the analyst and where lies, in the space that determines this position, the function of the partial object. (Lacan, 2014, pp. 93–94)

So, Lacan is reinterpreting the impasse of castration anxiety by saying that the analyst does not occupy the place of the guardian of castration but the place of the object that can on occasion cause anxiety.

We shan't do what we reproach all the others with doing, namely, to elide the analyst from the text of the experience we're examining. The anxiety unto which we have to bring a formula here is an anxiety that corresponds to us, an anxiety that we provoke, an anxiety with which we have on occasion a decisive relationship. (Lacan, 2014, p. 57)

If there is one analyst who was quite certain about the anxiety object of her analysands, and who advocated triggering then alleviating this anxiety through interpretations, that analyst is Melanie Klein. In her 1955 article "The psycho-analytic play technique: its history and significance", she declares the following on how she invented this technique with her first patient:

I deviated from some of the rules so far established, for I interpreted what I thought to be most urgent in the material the child presented to me and found my interest focusing on his anxieties and the defences against them. This new approach soon confronted me with serious problems. The anxieties I encountered when analysing this first case were very acute, and although I was strengthened in the belief that I was working on the right lines by observing the alleviation of anxiety again and again produced by my interpretations, I was at times perturbed by the intensity of the fresh anxieties which were being brought into the open. On one such occasion I sought advice from Dr Karl Abraham. He replied that since my interpretations up to then had often produced relief and the analysis was obviously progressing, he saw no ground for changing the method of approach. I felt encouraged by his support and, as it happened, in the next few days the child's anxiety, which had come to a head, greatly diminished, leading to further improvement. The conviction gained in this analysis strongly influenced the whole course of my analytic work. (Klein, 1975a, p. 123)

Here, therefore, we meet a first contrast between the certainty obtained by the practitioners of countertransference in their various imaginary experiences and the certainty that Melanie Klein snatches from anxiety. We may draw on Lacan's indications so as to read in these two contrasting approaches the effect of bringing the transference into play around the object *a*.

Betting on effects of speech or believing in cognitive processes

The certainty drawn from the anxiety at stake in Melanie Klein's technique was effectively transmitted in her school, despite the fact that contemporary Kleinians use countertransference in an adapted form under the name "projective identification". We meet an example of this today on the website of the *International Journal of Psycho-Analysis*. The site is currently hosting an interesting and lively debate in the wake of the journal's publication of a "psychoanalytic controversy" between an American ego-psychology psychoanalyst, Fred Busch, and the well-known London-based Kleinian analyst, Betty Joseph.

Under the title "A missing link in psychoanalytic technique: psychoanalytic consciousness", Busch expresses his surprise that what is so interesting for neurosciences, namely, consciousness, is not attracting interest amongst psychoanalysts, especially Kleinians. He takes up the Anna-Freudian flame and attacks the prestige of the unconscious in order to set out the virtues of approaching the defence mechanisms via the "surface" (Busch & Joseph, 2004). He takes his bearings from a mechanism of duplication between analyst and analysand that is analogous to (though slightly different from) the mechanism we have seen at work in the practitioners of countertransference. This duplication passes through to the analysand's interior. It occurs first between the brain and the world, since the mind is the reflection of the world by virtue of its cognitive processes. Thanks to consciousness, these processes can be meta-represented in a mirror that is dubbed "reflection". The unconscious is thus a mere cognitive process that is not yet conscious:

> It is my position that inherent in every interpretation of the unconscious in clinical psychoanalysis is an implied definition of psychoanalytic consciousness. Whenever we interpret something unknown to a patient we express our belief it is knowable. (Busch & Joseph, 2004, p. 567)

The technical criticism that Busch levels at the Kleinians is that they believe they are relieving anxiety by interpreting the deepest unconscious fantasies, when in fact one can only interpret those agencies that lie close to the surface based on a meaning that is accessible to the patient in his cognitive processes. Busch proposes objectifying them and duplicating them so as to enable them to be accessed, in spite of the emotions that inhibit the subject:

> [O]ne component of a psychoanalytic understanding of conscious-ness is a change in the patient's capacity to keep in mind and reflect upon his thinking. [...] With analysis we expect the patient to develop the potential for reflection. (Busch & Joseph, 2004, p. 568)

He specifies what he means by this:

> A patient may know he is angry with his boss (a perception of a feeling), but this is different than knowing *he* is angry with his boss. This latter type of "knowing" includes a conscious awareness that he is the source of his anger. We may make an interpretation to a patient that is deeply unconscious, and the patient may now "know" this about himself, but this is very different to the patient experiencing the interpretation as a way of knowing himself. To state it in its most pithy form, *psychoanalytic consciousness involves the potential for awareness of the role of one's own mind in effecting life in and outside of the analytic office.* Psychoanalytic consciousness is not a static form, but a highly variegated gradation, beginning with an inkling, a dim awareness, that there is a lot going on in one's mind. (Busch & Joseph, 2004, p. 569)

Busch's "variegated gradation" of consciousness is a direct borrow-ing from cognitivist vocabulary without taking any distance whatso-ever from this vocabulary. This is not the essential matter, however. The decisive point is that anxiety is being left by the wayside in favour of a much more vague category of "negative emotions". For Busch, everything is played out in the patient's mind, which has to stand up to these negative emotions as inhibitions in a cognitive process. Thus, fear is described as follows: "the fear in potentially knowing (a thought, a feeling) is what leads a patient into repetitive actions, while psycho-analysis can offer the possibility for reflection" (Busch & Joseph, 2004, p. 571). I am in agreement with François Leguil's analysis, which reads the collapse in the distinction between *fear* and *anxiety* as the key to the new cognitive psychology of the emotions (Leguil, 2005). Busch concludes his article by reproaching the Kleinians for not having an adequate theory of the ego, of its cognition of the unconscious, and for failing to differentiate it sufficiently from the "self".

Betty Joseph replies to Busch that what allows him to differentiate between the patient who subjectifies interpretations in analysis and the patient who considers them to be a knowledge that is foreign to his experience, as she expresses it, is transference: "to me the place where experience is experienced is in the relationship between patient and analyst—the transference" (Joseph, 2004, p. 573). Thus, what unites the two participants is above all projective identification. For Joseph, the transference is that which embodies what Busch calls "potential for reflection", to the extent that

> the analyst should be able to feel how he is being subjected to pressures from the patient and by becoming aware, not actually live them out […], but to use this awareness to help his understanding. (Joseph, 2004, p. 573)

Thus, she takes on board the opposition that Busch draws between *thinking* and *reflecting on one's thinking*, but she considers this transmutation to occur on the side of the analyst.

Betty Joseph's rejection of cognitive reflection and the reduction of the unconscious to neuronal processes inspires our sympathy, but her conception of the psychoanalyst in the locus of the Other does not adequately separate the two sides of transference. We can see this with the example that she puts to Busch of the way in which she deals with a patient whose sessions are repetitive and empty, and with whom none of her interpretations seem to give rise to anything really significant. The subject seems to be experiencing nothing in the sessions. Joseph reports a dream from the fourth year of treatment:

> *The patient was in a large place, something was going wrong; she was on one side of the place, the analyst on the other. I, the analyst, took it on myself to phone for help; my patient felt resigned and sad. She queried to herself would the phone call be helpful or make more trouble since the police might just burst in.* (Joseph, 2004, p. 574)

For Joseph, this dream describes perfectly the transferential atmosphere of the treatment: hope, mistrust, suspicion, and paranoid anxieties.

> From the point of view of the experiencing by both patient and analyst, this is very relevant since I am so frequently put in the position of either waiting and getting almost nowhere in the pauses and shifts, or feeling a desperate need to get on with things, to break in and disturb my patient's passivity and resignation. (Joseph, 2004, p. 574)

So, Joseph confides to the analysand her interpretation of "what is going on" as though it were what is effectively happening in the patient's head. Projective identification allows her to interpret the modality of the Other that the analysand constructs, along with the split objects that reside in this Other. In fact, here the analyst occupies the place of the omniscient narrator in the pre-Proust novel. Much as the objects have been described as partial and split, they are set within a whole. They are personified and embodied in each of the partners.

One of the participants in the online debate distances himself from Betty Joseph's interpretative certainty by noting that he is perplexed to read that an analyst of Joseph's calibre is always arriving at the same place with her patients, namely that the patient is said to be defending himself against some supposed dependence on her, while failing to allow the analyst to help him. It is my suspicion that this commentator is an analyst who has already been told something along these lines in supervision.

Busch replies that the dream in question shows above all that the analyst is not really speaking to her patient's surface-ego, she is too far away from it. This is why the patient calls her on the phone. This controversy on the nature of interpretation and the place of transference in treatment seems to be dominated by imaginary phenomena and the will to hold oneself at a distance from the dissymmetrical structure of the transferential phenomenon.

The place of the Other in the transference

The IPA website allows us to read all sorts of opinions in this controversy, with friends of one or the other on either side of the Atlantic offering a range of contributions. Mitchell Wilson contrasts Joseph's approach, in which the patient "does things to the analyst", with Busch's approach, where "the analyst does things to the patient". He declines to support either of them, saying, "what is lacking in this discussion is an essential theoretical reference point": Lacan's concept of dyadic or imaginary relationships. He makes reference to Lacan's L schema and the mirror stage, concluding with André Green's notion of the necessity of third-ness. Based in Berkeley California, Wilson reads Lacan through the writings of John P. Muller and he converses with Owen Renik (Wilson, 2003). His use of Lacanian reference points to designate the imaginary dimension represents a first step which we shall now pursue.

Betty Joseph's version of the analyst *knows what is at stake*, whereas Busch's version *tries to obtain from the patient himself an objective descrip-tion of the latter's thoughts*. Busch strives to obtain a sort of scientific per-spective. For us, this recalls the perspective that Lacan, in the *Anxiety* Seminar, sees at work in Thomas Szasz. Szasz posits that,

> the final end of any analysis, didactic or otherwise, can only be defined as the patient's initiation into a scientific point of view on his movements.
>
> [This is] the scientific point of view, inasmuch as its aim is always to consider lack as something that can be filled, in stark contrast to the problematic of an experience that includes within it the taking into account of lack as such. (Lacan, 2014, p. 145)[3]

Whether it be by dint of projective identification or scientific self-knowing, the subject-supposed-to-know here finds itself solidified and embodied in an agency. Nothing is missing here, and we can see how hard it is to situate the incompleteness of the Other.

We might say that within this perspective, transference has become real. Yet, as Jacques-Alain Miller underlines in the above-cited article, Lacan insists on the fact that "the subject-supposed-to-know is not real".

We need to lead our IPA colleagues further in their reference to Lacan. Then, they might be able not only to think about the imaginary relationships between analyst and analysand, not only about egoic objectifications, but also about the fact that "interpreting the transfer-ence amounts to filling an empty standstill by means of a lure" (Miller, 2003b).[4] This standstill, which is a zone in which the insistent signifiers overlap with the object *a*, is especially evident in the phenomenon of acting-out where what is involved is the demonstration of an unknown desire by means of an object that has become visible, a morsel of flesh abandoned to the Other. As Lacan puts it in the *Anxiety* Seminar:

The crux of what is on show is this remainder, this offcut, which falls away in the affair.

Betwixt the subject [...] and the Other, which cannot be authenticated, never fully authenticated, what emerges is the remainder, *a*, the pound of flesh. (Lacan, 2014, p. 124)

This pound of flesh accompanies the knowledge that is obtained in the experience:

[A]s soon as it becomes known, as soon as something comes to knowledge, something is lost and the surest way of approaching this lost something is to conceive of it as a bodily fragment. (Lacan, 2014, p. 134)

The analyst himself, if he has become the object *a* of the analysand's body, is then in a position to fall away or separate from the analysand. This is why Lacan turns to the example of Freud's case of the young homosexual woman.

[W]ith the young homosexual woman—which is a case where the function of the *a* is in a way so prevalent that it even went to the point of passing over into the real, a *passage à l'acte*, whose symbolic relation he nonetheless comprehends so well—Freud gives in. *I won't manage anything*, he tells himself, and he passes her on to a female colleague. He is the one who takes the initiative of *dropping* her. (Lacan, 2014, p. 113)

With this structuring of the *a* around the act of *letting drop*, Lacan allows us to think more carefully about what Melanie Klein approached with her primal object of envy, an object that is situated prior to repression. At the end of "Envy and gratitude", one of her last major texts (1957), Melanie Klein states that, for her, one has to target the defence that was erected prior to the onset of repression:

[I]n *Inhibition, Symptoms and Anxiety*, Freud had suggested that there may be methods of defence earlier than repression. [...]

As regards technique, I have attempted to show that by analysing over and over again the anxieties and defences bound up with envy and destructive impulses, progress in integration can be achieved. [...]

> I have found that the anxieties aroused by interpretations of hate
> and envy toward the primal object, and the feeling of persecution
> by the analyst whose work stirs up those emotions, are more painful
> than any other material we interpret. (Klein, 1975b, pp. 231–232)

In this way Melanie Klein accounts for the paradoxical phenomenon
that she meets in training analyses. The analysis might well have gone
on for some time, getting deeper and deeper, but one would invariably
come across a virulent anxiety and an eagerness to let the analyst drop,
which she calls "attacks on the analyst", on his work and thoughts.

Beyond this imaginary dimension specific to the object *a*, Lacan
accounts more fully for the way in which the partners turn around the
same pivotal point like the blades of a fan, a pivot that has the structure
of this *letting drop*:

> For who, in perceiving the two partners move like the two panels
> of a screen that swivels in my previous lines, cannot grasp that the
> transference has only ever been the pivotal hub of these very turns?
> (Lacan, 1995, p. 10)[5]

This structure is at work in the transferential relationships that tie Betty
Joseph's patient to her analyst, just as much as the paranoid anxieties
of persecution. This *letting drop*, here imaginarised in the montage of
acting-out, is read by Lacan as lying at the heart of the analytic experience, and as we are about to see it can denote the subject's relation to the
analytic discourse as a whole.

The roots of a symptom

The stark contrast between Betty Joseph's position and Busch's position
exposes the limitations of the dialectic processes of reconciliation that
Kernberg and Widlöcher are fond of constructing, just as the discussion
to which these positions have given rise gives us an idea of the monumental problem that is racking the IPA. This term has been used by
Renik who recently described the situation as follows:

> [W]e face a monumental problem because—as we well know—
> there is no consensus among us as to the *nature* of excellence in
> psychoanalytic work. What some of us will judge to be an analyst's
> creative and useful technical innovation, others of us will consider

irresponsible self-indulgence on the analyst's part; what some
of us will regard as an analyst's advisable caution and restraint,
others of us will see as the analyst's self-protective inhibition; what
impresses some of us as sensitive interpretation of the patient's
here-and-now experience, others will see as an avoidance of the
transference relationship and an impediment to the unfolding
of the patient's unconscious conflicts; what to some will seem
a timely reconstruction, others will perceive as an invitation to
intellectualise and ruminate about the past; and so on. (Renik, 2003,
p. 43/2005, p. 60)[6]

Having initially been played out around these two partisan polarities
with a central core of eager conciliators, the online discussion soon
shifted towards epistemic considerations due to the limitations of the
theoretical debates. This unease in psychoanalysis, a direct result of
uncertainty in the face of the act (an uncertainty that has seized hold of
this divided community), has given rise to an appeal and a false rem-
edy. Another of the stateside commentators on the website has pursued
the debate in symptomatic fashion by claiming that we know how the
same clinical material can be used to support different and contradictory theories, and that an apparent absence of methodology by which
to examine the various theoretical claims shows that analysts have
"failed". He laments the lack of internal resources to evaluate the divergent theories, but speaks favourably of how analysts have been led to
acknowledge the importance of databases that have been established
by the vast technological developments in the cognate professions: neu-
robiology, research on newborns, evolutionary theories, and so on.

The enthusiasm for cognate sciences that this author betrays allows
us to see a mechanism that is currently at work in the psychoanalytic
movement. The guilt at having "failed" is driving the movement into
the clutches of evaluative verifications. It is not just evaluative pressure
from public authorities that is pushing some psychoanalysts into evaluative and quantitative studies, in search of some impossible universal
measurement parameter.

We should not be weeping over the absence of empirical methodology, but rather grasping the shape that the anxiety of today's psychoanalyst is taking. The analyst's knowledge, which used to ground
the certainty of his act, is too fragmented to provide any support.
The humble and modest analyst, the contemporary of democratic
methodological incertitude, has lost his way and is ready to latch onto

any scientistic verification that is offered to him. Those in the IPA who refuse the intersubjective conception and the evaporation of the real of the unconscious that it brings about have been seeking refuge in the prestige and mirage of numerical figures and databases, and dreaming of filling the lack by means of science.

Now is the moment to conclude, with Lacan, that there are two inroads to the real, and that they are unconnected:

> [T]here is *either* the function of the concept as Hegel would have it, that is, the symbolic hold over the real, *or* the hold that we have, the one anxiety gives us, the sole final perception and as such the perception of all reality—and [...] between the two, one has to choose. (Lacan, 2014, p. 333)

Science is now bringing the Hegelian *concept* into realisation in its universal dimension. The analytic act on the other hand offers no other line of recourse but the potential to snatch certainty from anxiety through the act itself (Lacan, 2014, p. 77).

Failing this, the temptation is great among the psychoanalysts themselves to give in to their anxiety and let psychoanalysis drop. We hope, through our critical dialogue, to steer them away from this dead end and help them to uncover, with us, the proper channel by which to pass.

Notes

1. See the dialogue between Jean-Claude Rolland and Michel de M'Uzan at the Open Colloquium organised by the SPP on the theme of *Le travail psychanalytique*, 23–24 November 2002, at UNESCO, Paris, as reported by Herbert Wachsberger. Available at: www.oedipe.org/fr/actualites/colloquespp/colloquesppecf.
2. [*La pensée sauvage*, the title of the 1962 book by Claude Lévi-Strauss, has been translated as *The Savage Mind*. "Savage thought" is a more literal rendering. (Tr.)]
3. Lacan is commenting on Szasz, 1957.
4. This is an echo of Lacan's formula from the 1951 "Presentation on transference": "What then does it mean to interpret transference? Nothing but to fill the emptiness of this standstill with a lure" (Lacan, 2006, p. 184)
5. [Translation modified.]
6. Quoted by Samuel Stein in the online discussion.

The new pathways of loss in the DSM-5 impasse

The following lecture was delivered at the colloquium Qui a peur du DSM-5 ? *held at the Maison des Mines, Paris, on 12 October 2013.*

The publication of the DSM-5 in May 2013 was the occasion for debate and a taking of sides that allowed us to contemplate the end of an era for a clinic that had been dominated by the shadow of the *Diagnostic and Statistical Manual of Mental Disorders* project. This project harboured the vast ambition of producing a clinic of logical-positivist inspiration,[1] a clinic that set its sights on an artificial language to be imposed on clinicians with an eye to eliminating any imprecision, meaning-shifts, or misunderstandings. This classification aimed above all to rectify the imprecision of the Babel of clinical traditions in favour of a language that would afford a rigid designation of clinical categories that were imagined to be perfectly distinct, regardless of any irreducible "comorbidity" at the factual level. This will to univocity in clinical language was to be carried through by clinical definitions that were said to be "operational".[2]

The logical form chosen by the DSM is that of a formal tree that classifies mental illnesses in keeping with the "botanical" model of genera, species and sub-species that was first presented by Linnaeus in his

Systema Naturae and later adopted by Darwin. The epistemologist Ian Hacking considers that the "fatal flaw" in the DSM project stems from this point of departure which has never been put in question and which remains unexamined within the system. There is no more reason for mental illnesses to fall within a botanical classification than there would be for the chemical elements that arise from a "periodic table". The periodic table has nothing botanical about it whatsoever. Hacking offers a deep-reaching critique: "Perhaps in the end the DSM will be regarded as a *reductio ad absurdum* of the botanical project in the field of insanity" (Hacking, 2013, p. 8).

The elements that were supposed to find an inscription within the classificatory tree needed to be the most univocal and straightforward possible so as to respond to the ambitions of the project. This was the aim that set the stage for the encounter between the DSM project and the cognitive-behavioural project. Directly observable elementary clinical items that had been reduced to symptoms that lay outside any broader clinical entity or seemingly senseless patterns of behaviour, fit perfectly with this positivist and botanical project of classification. In this respect, even though the DSM project cannot be reduced to its cognitive-behavioural dimension, it cannot be separated from it either.

This point of departure was never to be examined again. Spitzer's DSM-III project in the 1970s drew its inspiration from psychologists' refinements in statistics so as to pitch the psychiatric clinic at the level of the most recent statistical requirements. The stress was put on techniques that would allow for solid "inter-rater reliability", that is, the fact of zero possible variation across the description of observed phenomena. The DSM's "atheoretical" classification was to prove to be increasingly based on a theory of statistics. Clinical questions *per se* were soon to be drowned out by questions of statistical technique.[3]

In this sense, the DSM project bears the stamp of a power grab in the clinical field by researchers over practitioners. This ascendancy held greater and greater sway for the thirty years over which the DSM project extended its reach. In their quest for a perfect language, the researchers sought to rectify all the "bad habits" of practitioners. At the end of the process, one can now say that with the DSM-5 the break between research and clinicians is complete. This is what Thomas Insel, director of the National Institute of Mental Health in the US, observed in a momentous announcement on 29 April 2013, a fortnight prior to the release of the DSM-5. He sees few variations between the DSM-IV-R and version 5. The latest version of the dictionary that had been organising the field of psychopathology conserved both its strength and its weakness. Its strength is its "inter-rater reliability". Its weakness remains its lack of "scientific validity". In other words, the language is perfect but it means nothing to the extent that its declared purpose is to measure something other than itself. Insel notes that the DSM is based on "a consensus about clusters of symptoms" that can be easily spotted, and not on the "objective" measure of anything whatsoever (Insel, 2013). This is why over the last two years the NIMH has been launching a project that is very dif-ferent from the DSM-5. It has been pooling together "research domain criteria" (RDoC) that include all the elements that have been isolated by research into objective signs in the field of psychopathology: neu-ro-imagery, likely biomarkers, alterations in cognitive function, and objectifiable neurological circuits across the three registers of cogni-tion, emotion, and behaviour. The collecting and assembling of these elements is performed without any regard for commonly accepted clinical categories, which they think of as mere surface effects. "This is why the NIMH will be re-orienting its research away from DSM cat-egories," writes Insel, "going forward, we will be supporting research projects that look across current categories". Once the initial aston-ishment was over, the damage-control spin got underway without a moment's ado. On 13 May, just prior to the opening of the American Psychiatric Association's annual congress, its new president, Jeffrey Lieberman, issued a joint statement with Insel on DSM-5 and RDoC, assuring us, needless to say, that both projects held their own specific relevance (Insel & Lieberman, 2013).

Efforts to get clinicians to change their mindset have been around for a while. Steven E. Hyman MD, current director of the Stanley Center for Psychiatric Research at the Broad Institute of MIT and Harvard, and former director of the NIMH from 1996 to 2001, was the first to advo-cate the necessity of opening up the DSM and the ICD to recent contri-butions from imaging, genetics and the neurosciences. Since Hyman, each of the successive NIMH directors has maintained this orienta-tion. The question, therefore, is why they waited so long to split away from the DSM system and to make such a clean break. My hypothesis is that the process of drafting the new DSM over the last fifteen years revealed that the contradictions at the heart of psychiatry were insolu-ble from the standpoint of the hardliners. Open opposition from the former architects of the DSM-III (Robert Spitzer) and IV (Allen Frances) to the orientations chosen by the DSM-5 Task Force culminated, as of 2009, in a series of open letters and complaints to the ruling bodies of the APA. The will to extend the categories to infra-clinical thresholds, to stigmatised "at risk" populations, in an ever-greater medicalisation of existence, threw the profession as a whole into a state of wide alert. The mounting conflicts of interest between universities and laboratory-financed researchers harmed the scientific credibility of opinion leaders in the psychiatric field whilst great disappointment with the actual benefits of the most recent generation of drugs, which were nevertheless presented as miracle solutions, served to undermine the benchmark measure of randomised clinical trials.

The previous APA congress in March 2012 was the occasion for the final round of negotiations. On the table was a proposition to drop the most criticised categories and to reduce the diverging discrepancies in the calculations for consequences of new drugs on different populations. This was to be in exchange for the green light to go to print issued by the higher echelons of the association. These negotiations met their goal. By December, the last commissions had weighed up all the potential consequences and printing got underway in January. Set at the steep price of $200 for the hardback edition and $140 in paperback, the volume was ready to be distributed far and wide thanks to a major logistical effort. The depreciation of the enterprise following Insel's announcement was massive and brutal.

The NIMH now wants to attach its project to the Obama administration's BRAIN Initiative research into cerebral functioning and modelling. This brain modelling is, however, still in its infancy. John Horgan at *Scientific American* sums up the lie of the land by saying that we are in a situation that "resembles genetics before the discovery of the double helix".[4] The field lacks any organising principle and so we are a long way from being able to tie the various biological clues to the different clinical levels open to observation. Three decades of the DSM project have failed to introduce any meaningful discoveries, but the RDoC scientific project which is supposed to be taking up the baton remains up in the air. Condemning the DSM project's lack of scientific pertinence does not change the fact that there is nothing to replace it. The break that has thereby been brought about between research and clinic effectively cuts the clinicians loose. They remain on their own, without any support from the ground of science.

The impasse of the DSM project is culminating in the evacuation of "clinical types" in favour of chimeras that drift off into the empyrean of calculus. Only *abandonment* remains: the abandonment of patients faced with the growing scarcity of credits allocated to a psychiatry that is considered to be increasingly costly; and the abandonment of an ever-larger population who end up on the street, in jail, or on excessive quantities of medication. This clinic of the abandonment of those who are all alone is relayed by the relentless surveillance of populations who are being left to their own devices in this way. The present-day relevance of Orwell's Big Brother is ever more astonishing, and teaches us the degree to which we are watched, listened in on, and recorded, thanks to the phenomenal processing power at the disposal of health and safety bureaucracies that are becoming more fully integrated as time goes on. Google, the eponymous enterprise dedicated to the digitalisation of the world, is being revealed as a partner of choice for the US administration in every aspect of the construction of our "digital future" (see Schmidt & Cohen, 2013).

Whilst the DSM instrument has not given rise to any discoveries, it has proven itself to be a mighty instrument for population management, assigning subjects to tick-boxes that can be processed ever-more efficiently by administrative language, then widening the administrative use of these categories beyond the healthcare field to include the spheres of insurance, social rights, and law. This extension, which was first seen in the US, has now gone global. As an instrument of management, it meets its limitations, even its failure, in the creation of inflationary bubble categories into which subjects are slotted, or even seek to be slotted. The assigning of subjects to different categories can be computed by healthcare bureaucracies, but the uses and wishes of those who find themselves assigned to them are unpredictable. Thus, there are constant shifts that in turn give rise to a particular kind of "slippery-soap effect".[5]

Next, when managers seek to reduce statistically observable "epidemics" by modifying their defining criteria, they come up against the wishes of the subjects themselves who might want, for example, to be considered "hyperactive" between thirty-three and forty-five years of age so as to be prescribed amphetamines (Cabut, 2013); or who might want to be considered "bipolar" because this label is less stigmatising than others; or who might even want to be considered "Asperger" so as to have access to special education programmes.

This kind of disoriented classificatory reshaping produces contradictory effects. Dropping pathological classifications for most of the behaviours that were considered sexually deviant at the start of the last century is going hand in hand with a pathologisation of manifold aspects of everyday life, right down to the most commonplace emotions. The constant and ongoing extension of the domain of depression is one of the most striking examples, but limits between normal and pathological are collapsing across the board.

The overly descriptive character of the clinical categories inherited from the clinic of the gaze, which have since been invalidated by science, are being referred to a continuum with those organic processes that are expected to be objectifiable at some future date, in keeping with the model of dementia processes that will evolve for upwards of fifteen years before finding an observable clinical translation. Instead of categories that can lead to belief in false distinctions, the researchers prefer a model that privileges continuity. The flipside of the "medicalisation of everyday life" process is precisely the recognition that "psychiatric patients are merely people who are a little less 'normal' than the rest" (Demazeux, 2013, p. 327). In its difficulty to set down the limits between normal and pathological, the DSM-5 is confirming in its own way that "everybody is mad, i.e. everyone is delusional" (Lacan, 2013), but within a clinic that forecloses the subject with no possibility of return. In the stead of the subject, we find "personality disorders" that have been reformatted and given a psychological cast by using complex matrices of "personality traits", revamped "characterologies" or "temperaments", and a seamless integration of symptoms and personalities. The new DSM has shrunk back from the enormity of this task, simply confining all of this to an appendix. These makeshift throw-togethers that maintain on the horizon a description of pathology in terms of "excesses of personality" remind us that the pathology of excess is particularly in step with the way that our era is experiencing the drive as mediated by the superego. The absence of the limits that used to provide the subject with firm identifications is leading all identifications to become both fluid and particularly sensitive to the command "Enjoy!" Limitlessness is thus the index of a world falling under the superego's sway. The subject finds himself all on his own having to cope with this "push towards jouissance". The extension of the clinic of addictions vouches for this.

What lies ahead of us is going to break entirely from any clinic of the subject and any sociological clinic, which the DSM still was. The contradictions will be strong between the ambition for "validity" with respect to a real that is targeted and the small share of effectivity (*Wirklichkeit*) that will be produced. The field of the neurosciences and that of the BRAIN Initiative are not unified by a common paradigm. As the likes of Horgan have put it, this does indeed look like the field of genetics prior to the discovery of the double helix. Hypotheses of strict biological determination are heavy with potential social stigma. How they are handled in the clinical field will necessarily imply the involvement of affected populations. Associating legal rights with the irreversible label that follows from each diagnosis presupposes considerable financing and a recasting of the healthcare system, as we are seeing for autism. The many bodies of administrative supervision that distribute healthcare in the US, the private insurance firms, and the complex Obamacare plan, are going to have to look long and hard if they are to appreciate fully the consequences of this in-between period.

In Europe, with the exception of the UK, the situation is characterised by a certain silence from university academics who have generally fallen in step behind the DSM without making their presence felt. Their discourse is more centralised than in the US. The double issue of the newspaper *Libération* from 8–9 May gave a good account of this. Bruno Falissard, an "epidemiologist and psychiatrist", is not all that dissatisfied with the DSM, leaving it to the Americans and their "societal difference". He stresses that the French clinic is, fortunately, "more phenomenological and closer to the subjective experience of patients". From his atypical position, he warns against such large-scale classificatory projects and fascination for vast series of statistics. "We've gone too far down the road of evidence-based medicine," says Falissard, "this medicine reliant on statistical studies concerns an [abstract] 'average' patient". He asks that greater attention be paid to singularity. In the meantime, the DSM remains the only classification system that holds any authority in the universities. It is on the side of clinicians that a boycott movement has taken shape. *Libération* journalist Éric Favereau also interviewed Patrick Landman, president of the collective Stop DSM-5, which groups together practitioners from the entirety of the clinical field. Their goal is to stop using the DSM in favour of the ICD recognised by the World Health Organization or to campaign for the French

Classification for Child and Adolescent Mental Disorders (CFTMEA), which the WHO considers to be too subjective.

In the UK, academics have not been gagged as they have on the continent. The dissident voices of Germán Berrios in Cambridge and David Healy at Cardiff University have been heard. The British Psychological Association has long sided against the biological and statistical orientation of the DSM, and it played a part in the campaign to boycott the manual with an open letter that drew wide support. On 13 May, the eve of the release of the DSM-5, the association's division of clinical psychology declared that it would be calling for a paradigm shift in mental health issues. It reiterated that

> psychiatric diagnosis is often presented as an objective statement of fact, but is, in essence, a clinical judgement based on observation and interpretation of behaviour and self-report, and thus subject to variation and bias.[6]

So it is that they maintain that mental health problems should be thought about above all in psychological and social terms.

Opposition to the DSM project and the system's internal contradictions mean that most likely there will not be any DSM-6 for a long while to come, and the clinical project will have to be rethought from scratch. The RDoC project, though it is still a dream of the NIMH, remains a project that subverts no less the traditional form of the cognitive-behavioural compromise. Certainly the project will seek to integrate the alteration of cognitive functions and their objectifiable circuits across the three essential domains of cognition, emotion, and behaviour, but the RDoC has the goal of mapping the entirety of these aspects across the continuum of the field, bypassing the DSM's various labels and sub-groups that endlessly sub-divide, and likewise bypassing an approach based on behavioural observation alone. The search for an "objectification" of cognitive functions in neuronal circuits that can be observed through imaging implies breaking off from an observation of human conduct that reduces it to mere lines of behaviour. Behaviour will be admitted into the new project only on the condition that it corresponds to the functioning of an observable neural circuit, but we are still a long way from being able to "objectify" behaviours that draw on the body as a whole, such as sitting on a chair, for instance. If you put someone under a positron camera and ask him simply to associate "to sit" with the word "chair", the number of zones that light up and are mobilised just to utter "I'm sitting on a chair" is immense. When it comes to more complicated conversations, the number is practically incalculable, for example, when the subject doesn't know which chair or when he is instructed not to sit on the chair that is being shown. These mechanisms introduce a sum of information that makes one marvel at just how it can be deployed in real-time conversation. One can only wonder as to the whereabouts of the integrating centre that would allow for these zones that treat the information associated with "sitting on a chair" to be unified so as to perform the action, not to mention when a slip of the tongue, a play on words, or a witticism is uttered when one is speaking. Furthermore, the Harvard-based Nobel laureate David Hubel has objected that

> this surprising tendency for attributes such as form, colour and movement to be handled by separate structures in the brain immediately raises the question of how all the information is finally assembled, say, for perceiving a bouncing red ball. It obviously must be assembled [...] [but where] and how, we have no idea. (Hubel, 1995, quoted in Le Fanu, 2010)

From our current standpoint, what we have learnt about the brain's functioning suggests that within the coming decade we shall know more about how it works and perhaps in detail that we can scarcely imagine at present, but we can also say that a certain number of fundamental points bearing on subjectivity will remain enigmatic. How will the cognitive-behavioural programme be modified? We shall see, but we can be sure that a good many different patchwork solutions will be put forward to save it.

The end of an era always brings with it peculiar jolts and jerks. We are emerging from a period in which a predominant paradigm was established that only allowed for opposition on the fringes. Now the entire field is shot through with fresh contradictions between scientific hardliners, public and private healthcare bureaucracies, upholders of various clinical traditions, and those appealing for a clinic of the subject. The cards are going to be reshuffled and the divergent interests of the different players are not about to converge in an overhauled unifying paradigm anytime soon. Something new will remain "lost in cognition". We shall continue to assume responsibility for the ongoing commentary of this loss.

Notes

1. As was noted by the author of *Qu'est-ce que le DSM?* who was in the main in favour of it. See Demazeux, 2013.
2. Already in 1955, Lacan was mocking the use of the word "op-er-a-tion-al" as an attempt to get rid of the rational, especially with respect to the use of operational criteria in ego psychology. See Lacan, 2006, p. 350.
3. This point was carefully noted back in 1992 by Stuart A. Kirk and Herb Kutchins (Kirk & Kutchins, 1992).
4. On his blog hosted by *Scientific American*, Horgan posted an article bearing the title "Psychiatry in crisis! Mental health director rejects psychiatric 'bible' and replaces with … nothing" (4 May, 2013).
5. On the "slippery standard" see Kirk and Kutchins, 1992, pp. 171–177.
6. Division of Clinical Psychology, "Position statement on the classification of behaviour and experience in relation to functional psychiatric diagnoses" (final version), 2013, p. 3.

REFERENCES

Ablon, J. S., & Jones, E. E. (2002). Validity of controlled clinical trials of psychotherapy: findings from the NIMH treatment of depression collaborative research program. *American Journal of Psychiatry, 159* (5): 775–783. Available at: ajp.psychiatryonline.org.

Aflalo, A. (2014). *The Failed Assassination of Psychoanalysis* (translated by A. R. Price). London: Karnac.

Allemand, L. (2004). Il y a 75, 000 ans, les premiers bijoux. *La Recherche, 375*: 47.

American Psychiatric Association (1994). *Diagnostic and Statistical Manual of Mental Disorders, DSM-IV*. Washington DC:APA.

Anon (2006a). The Omega point. *The Economist*, 19 January: 72.

Anon (2006b). Learning without learning. *The Economist*, 21 September: 78–79.

Ansermet, F., & Magistretti, P. J. (2007). *Biology of Freedom: Neural Plasticity, Experience and the Unconscious* (translated by S. Fairfield). London: Karnac.

Ansermet, F., & Magistretti, P. J. (2008). Neuronal plasticity: a new paradigm for resilience. *Schweizer Archiv für Neurologie und Psychiatrie, 159* (8): 475–479.

Arnal, S., & Sibony, D. (2005). Freud cloué au pilori. *L'Hebdo* (Lausanne), 13 October, *41*.

Atran, S. (2002). *In Gods We Trust: The Evolutionary Landscape of Religion*. Oxford: Oxford University Press.

Atran, S. (2003). Théorie cognitive de la culture; une alternative évolutionniste à la sociobiologie et à la sélection collective. *L'Homme, 166*: 107–143.

Atran, S. (2004). Origine et évolution de la culture humaine. Paper delivered at the Conference *Origine de l'homme et souffrance psychique*, Institut des Sciences Cognitives, Lyon, 6 November.

Aubert, J. (2005). Ego nominor N … ego. *La lettre mensuelle, 240*: 52–56.

Aubert, J. (2010). *Passed over* stories (translated by A. R. Price). *Hurly-Burly, 4*: 167–184.

Benkimoun, P. (2004). Le vrai et le faux des omega-3. *Le Monde*, 31 March, p. 26.

Bennett, M. R., & Hacker, P. M. S. (2003). *Philosophical Foundations of Neuroscience*. Malden, MA: Blackwell.

Blackburn, S. (1998). Wittgenstein, Wright, Rorty and minimalism. *Mind, 107*: 157–181. Reprinted in S. Blackburn & K. Simmons (Eds.), *Truth* (1999). Oxford: Clarendon Press.

Bliss, T. V. P., & Lømo, T. (1973). Long-lasting potentiation of synaptic transmission in the dentate area of the anesthetized rabbit following stimulation of the perforant path. *The Journal of Physiology, 232*: 331–356.

Bollas, C. (1987). Expressive uses of the countertransference: notes to the patient from oneself. Chapter Twelve of *The Shadow of the Object*. New York: Columbia University Press.

Borenstein, D. (2001). Evidence-based psychiatry. *Psychiatric News*, May, *36*: 3.

Botella, S., & Botella, C. (2005). *The Work of Psychic Figurability: Mental States Without Representation* (translated by A. Weller). New York: Brunner-Routledge.

Brooks, D. (2005). Psst! Human capital. *New York Times*, 13 November, p. 12.

Brusset, B. (2004). Sur le problème de la réglementation des psychothérapies. Posted on the website of the Société psychanalytique de Paris, 10 March.

Busch, F., & Joseph, B. (2004). A missing link in psychoanalytic technique: psychoanalytic consciousness. *International Journal of Psycho-Analysis, 85*: 567–572.

Cabut, S. (2013). Hyperactivité: la ritaline est-elle mal prescrite? *Le Monde (Science & Médecine)*, 19 June, p. 2.

Carey, B. (2004). Pills or talk? If you're confused, no wonder. *The New York Times*, 8 June.

Carey, B. (2005). Antidepressant safety may include adult patients. *The New York Times*, 18 February.

Caroli, F. (2005). Psychopathie: genèse et évolution clinique. HAS, *Prise en charge de la psychopathie*, pp. 14–15.

Carroll, L. (1865). *Alice's Adventures in Wonderland*. London: Macmillan [various reprints available].

Castellucci, V., Pinsker, H., Kupfermann, I., & Kandel, E. R. (1970). Neuronal mechanisms of habituation and dishabituation of the gill-withdrawal reflex in aplysia. *Science, 167*: 1745–1748.

Chomsky, N. (1971). The case against B. F. Skinner. *New York Review of Books,* 30 December, 18–24.

Cialdella, P. (2007). Réponse à Perron et al. concernant leur texte: "Quelques remarques méthodologiques à propos du rapport de l'Inserm *Psychothérapie, trois approches évaluées*". *L'Encéphale, 33* (5): 783–790.

Cipriani, A., Barbui, C., & Geddes, J. R. (2005). Suicide, depression, and antidepressants: patients and clinicians need to balance benefits and harms. *British Medical Journal, 330* (7488): 373–374.

Clinton, H. (2003). *Living History*. New York: Simon & Schuster.

Damasio, A. (2004). *Looking For Spinoza: Joy, Sorrow, and the Feeling Brain*. San Diego, CA: Harcourt.

Demazeux, S. (2013). *Qu'est-ce que le DSM?* Paris: Éditions d'Ithaque.

Denzin, N. K., & Lincoln, V. S. (2000). *Handbook of Qualitative Research*. Thousand Oaks, CA: Sage.

Dupuy, J. -P. (2000). *On the Origins of Cognitive Science: The Mechanization of the Mind* (translated by M. B. DeBevoise). Princeton, NJ: Princeton University Press [reprinted Cambridge MA: MIT, 2009].

Eco, U. (1995). *The Search for the Perfect Language* (translated by J. Fentress). Oxford: Blackwell.

Engel, P., & Rorty, R. (2007). *What's the Use of Truth?* (translated by W. McCuaig). New York: Columbia University Press.

Fodor, J. (1975). *The Language of Thought*. Cambridge, MA: Harvard University Press.

Fodor, J. (1983). *The Modularity of Mind: An Essay on Faculty Psychology*. Cambridge, MA: MIT.

Fodor, J. (1987). Modules, frames, fridgeons, sleeping dogs, and the music of the spheres. In: J. Garfield (Ed.), *Modularity in Knowledge Representation and Natural-Language Understanding* (pp. 25–36). Cambridge, MA: MIT.

Fonagy, P., Gergely, G., Jurist, E. L., & Target, M. (2002). *Affect Regulation, Mentalisation and the Development of the Self*. New York: Other.

Freud, S. (1895a). A Project for a Scientific Psychology (translated by J. Strachey). *S. E., 1*. London: Hogarth.

Freud, S. (1895b). On the Grounds for Detaching a Particular Syndrome from Neurasthenia under the Description "Anxiety Neurosis" (translated by J. Rickman). *S. E., 3*. London: Hogarth.

Freud, S. (1920g). Beyond the Pleasure Principle (translated by J. Strachey). *S. E., 18*. London: Hogarth.

Freud, S. (1925h). Negation (translated by J. Riviere). *S. E., 19*. London: Hogarth.

Freud, S. (1926d). *Inhibitions, Symptoms and Anxiety* (translated by A. Strachey). *S. E., 20*. London: Hogarth.

Freud, S. (1930a). *Civilisation and its Discontents* (translated by J. Riviere). *S. E., 21*. London: Hogarth.

Freud, S. (1987). Overview of the transference neuroses [1915] (translated by A. Hoffer & P. T. Hoffer). In: I. Grubrich-Simitis (Ed.), *A Phylogenetic Fantasy: Overview of the Transference Neuroses* (pp. 1–72). Cambridge, MA: Harvard University Press.

Fulford, K. W. M. (2004). Facts/values; ten principles of values-based medicine. In: J. Radden (Ed.), *The Philosophy of Psychiatry: A Companion* (pp. 205–234). New York: Oxford University Press.

Gibbons, M., Limoges, C., Nowotny, H., Schwartzman, S., Scott, P., & Trow, M. (1994). *The New Production of Knowledge: the Dynamics of Science and Research in Contemporary Societies*. London: Sage.

Gilpin, K. N. (2004). Spitzer sues, accusing Glaxo of fraud. *International Herald Tribune*, 3 June.

Grissom, R. J. (1996). The magical number 7 +/− 2: meta-meta-analysis of the probability of superior outcome in comparisons involving therapy, placebo and control. *Journal of Consulting and Clinical Psychology, 64* (5): 973–982.

Hacking, I. (2004a). Minding the brain. *New York Review of Books, 51* (11): 35–36.

Hacking, I. (2004b). Mindblind. *London Review of Books, 26* (20): 15–16.

Hacking, I. (2013). Lost in the forest. *London Review of Books, 35* (15): 7–8.

Halpern, S. (2006). Thanks for the memory. *New York Review of Books, 53* (15).

Harris, G. (2004). Mix of drugs and therapy found best for depressed teenagers. *International Herald Tribune*, 3 June.

Haute Autorité de santé (2005). *Prise en charge de la psychopathie*, public hearing on 15–16 December, Paris. Available at: www.anaes.fr.

Holden, S. (2002). Taking to a gullible world like a mouse to Swiss cheese. *The New York Times (Arts Section)*, 25 December, p. 1.

Horgan, J. (2013). Psychiatry in crisis! mental health director rejects psychiatric "bible" and replaces with ... nothing. Posted on blog hosted by *Scientific American*, 4 May.

Hubel, D. (1995). *Eye, Brain and Vision*. New York: Scientific American Library.

Hugnet, G. (2004). *Antidépresseurs: la grande intoxication, ce que 5 millions de patients ne savent pas encore*. Paris: Le cherche midi.

Insel, T. R. (2013). Transforming diagnosis. Posted on *Director's Blog* at: www.nimh.nih.gov/about/director/2013/transforming-diagnosis.shtml.

Insel, T. R., & Lieberman, J. A. (2013). DSM-5 and RDoC: shared interests. Available at: www.nimh.nih.gov/news/science-news/2013/dsm-5-and-rdoc-shared-interests.shtml.

Inserm Collective (2002). *Troubles mentaux: Dépistage et prévention chez les enfants et l'adolescent*. Paris: Éditions de l'Inserm.

Inserm Collective (2004). *Psychothérapie: trois approches évaluées*. Paris: Éditions de l'Inserm.

Inserm Collective (2005). *Trouble des conduites chez l'enfant et l'adolescent*. Paris: Éditions de l'Inserm.

Jacob, P. (2004). Origine de l'esprit humain et théorie de l'esprit. Paper delivered at the conference *Origine de l'homme et souffrance psychique*, Institut des Sciences Cognitives, Lyon, 6 November.

Joseph, B. (2004). Rejoinder. *The International Journal of Psycho-Analysis, 85*: 572–574.

Kagan, R. (2002). Power and weakness. *Policy Review, 113*: 3–2.

Kaltenthaler, E., Shackley, P., Stevens, K., Beverley, C., Parry, G., & Chilcott, J. (2002). A systematic review and economic evaluation of computerised cognitive behaviour therapy for depression and anxiety. *Health Technology Assessment, 6* (22).

Kamin, L. J. (1969). Predictability, surprise, attention, and conditioning. In: B. A. Campbell & R. M. Church (Eds.), *Punishment and Aversive Behaviour* (pp. 279–296). New York: Appleton-Century-Crofts.

Kandel, E. R. (1999). Biology and the future of psychoanalysis: a new intellectual framework for psychiatry revisited. *American Journal of Psychiatry, 156*: 505–524.

Kandel, E. R. (2006). *In Search of Memory: the Emergence of a New Science of Mind*. New York: Norton.

Kendell, R., & Jablensky, A. (2003). Distinguishing between the validity and utility of psychiatric diagnoses. *American Journal of Psychiatry, 160*: 4–12.

Kirk, S. A., & Kutchins, H. (1992). *The Selling of DSM: The Rhetoric of Science in Psychiatry*. New Brunswick: Aldine Transaction.

Klein, M. (1975a). The psycho-analytic play technique: its history and significance [1955]. In: *Envy and Gratitude and Other Works 1946–1963* (pp. 122–140). London: Hogarth.

Klein, M. (1975b). Envy and gratitude [1957]. In *Envy and Gratitude and Other Works 1946–1963* (pp. 176–235). London: Hogarth.

Knight, R. P. (1941). Evaluation of the results of psychoanalytic therapy. *American Journal of Psychiatry, 98*: 434–446.

Krugman, P. (2005). Pride, prejudice, insurance. *New York Times*, 7 November.

Kupiec, J. -J., & Sonigo, P. (2000). *Ni Dieu ni gène: Pour une autre théorie de l'hérédité*. Paris: Seuil.

Lacan, J. (1974). Freud per sempre; intervista con Jacques Lacan. *Panorama*, 21 November.

Lacan, J. (1977a). Intervention lors des conférences du champ freudien, 9 mars 1976. *Analytica, 4*: 16–18.

Lacan, J. (1977b). *The Seminar of Jacques Lacan Book XI: The Four Fundamental Concepts of Psychoanalysis* (translated by A. Sheridan). New York: Norton, 1998.

Lacan, J. (1988). *The Seminar of Jacques Lacan Book II: The Ego in Freud's Theory and in the Technique of Psychoanalysis, 1954–1955* (translated by S. Tomaselli). Cambridge: Cambridge University Press.

Lacan, J. (1995). Proposition of 9 October 1967 on the Psychoanalyst of the School (translated by R. Grigg). *Analysis, 6*: 1–13.

Lacan, J. (1998a). *The Seminar of Jacques Lacan Book XX: On Feminine Sexuality, the Limits of Love and Knowledge (Encore), 1972–1973* (translated by B. Fink). New York: Norton.

Lacan, J. (1998b). *Le séminaire livre V: Les formations de l'inconscient, 1957–1958*. Paris: Seuil.

Lacan, J. (2001a). La méprise du sujet supposé savoir [1967]. In: *Autres écrits* (pp. 329–339). Paris: Seuil.

Lacan, J. (2001b). … *ou pire*; Compte rendu du séminaire, 1971–1972 [1975]. In: *Autres écrits* (pp. 547–552). Paris: Seuil.

Lacan, J. (2005a). *Le séminaire livre XXIII: Le sinthome, 1975–1976*. Paris: Seuil.

Lacan, J. (2005b). Discours aux Catholiques [1960]. In: *Le Triomphe de la Religion, précédé de Discours aux Catholiques* (pp. 9–66). Paris: Seuil.

Lacan, J. (2006). *Écrits: The First Complete Edition in English* (translated by B. Fink, R. Grigg & H. Fink). New York: Norton.

Lacan, J. (2013). There are four discourses … (translated by A. R. Price). *Culture/Clinic*, Spring, 1.

Lacan, J. (2014). *The Seminar Book X: Anxiety, 1962–1963* (translated by A. R. Price). Cambridge: Polity.

Lambert, M. J. (2003). *Bergin and Garfield's Handbook of Psychotherapy and Behavior Change* (5th edn). New York: Wiley.

Laroche, S. (2001). Neuro-modelage des souvenirs. *La Recherche—La mémoire et l'oubli, 344*: 20–24.

Laroche, S. (2006). Comment les neurones stockent les souvenirs? *Les dossiers de la Recherche, 22*: 29–30.

Laurent, D. (2004). Du désir de standardisation massive. Posted on the website www.forumpsy.org on 26 March; published in *Letterina*, 2005, *38*: 11–19.

Laurent, D. (2005). Les redresseurs de gènes et le tort fait au social. *La Cause freudienne*, *61*: 23–27.

Le Fanu, J. (2010). Science's dead end. *Prospect*, 21 July. Available at: www.prospectmagazine.co.uk/magazine/sciences-dead-end/#. UrFyymRdWp0.

Leguil, F. (2005). Le stade de l'angoisse. *La Cause freudienne*, *59*: 23–32.

Lesourd, S. (2005). Psychopathie: genèse et évolution clinique. Psychopathies et normes sociales. HAS, *Prise en charge de la psychopathie*, pp. 16–18.

Leuzinger-Bohleber, M., Stuhr, U., Rüger, B., & Beutel, M. (2003). How to study the "quality of psychoanalytic treatments" and their long-term effects on patients' well-being. A representative, multi-perspective follow-up study. *International Journal of Psycho-Analysis*, *84* (2): 263–290.

Luborsky, L., Rosenthal, R., Diguer, L., Andrusyna, T. P., Berman, J. S., Levitt, J. T., Seligman, D. A., & Krause, E. D. (2002). The dodo bird verdict is alive and well—mostly. *Clinical Psychology: Science and Practice*, *9* (1): 2–12.

Luminet, J. -P. (2008). *The Wraparound Universe* (translated by E. Novak). Natick, MA: Peters.

Marcelli, D., & Cohen, D. (2005). Outils d'évaluation chez l'enfant et l'adolescent: la psychopathie. HAS, *Prise en charge de la psychopathie*, pp. 25–30.

March, J. S., Silva, S., Petrycki, S., Curry, J., Wells, K., Fairbank, J., Burns, B., Domino, M., McNulty, S., Vitiello, B., & Severe, J. (2004). Fluoxetine, cognitive-behavioral therapy, and their combination for adolescents with depression: treatment for adolescents with depression study (TADS) randomized controlled trial. *Journal of American Medical Association*, *292* (7): 807–820.

Marr, D. (1982). *Vision: A Computational Investigation into the Human Representation and Processing of Visual Information*. New York: Freeman [reprinted Cambridge, MA: MIT, 2010].

McKibbin, R. (2006). The destruction of the public sphere. *London Review of Books*, *28* (1): 3–6.

Messer, S. B. (2002). Empirically supported treatments: cautionary notes. *Medscape General Medicine*, *4* (4). Available at: www.medscape.com.

Miller, J. -A. (1997). Un réel pour la psychanalyse. *La Lettre mensuelle*, *161*: 25–28.

Miller, J. -A. (1998). The seminar of Barcelona on *Die Wege der Symptombildung* (translated by R. Barros). *Psychoanalytical Notebooks of the London Circle*, *1*: 11–65.

Miller, J. -A. (2000). ... *du nouveau*, Paris: Huysmans.

Miller, J. -A. (2003a). Une incroyable exaltation. In: *Lakant* (pp. 27–40). Paris: Rue Huysmans Collection/Navarin-Seuil.

Miller, J. -A. (2003b). Countertransference and intersubjectivity (translated by B. P. Fulks). *Lacanian Ink, 22*: 8–53.

Miller, J. -A. (2005). *The Pathology of Democracy. A Letter to Bernard Accoyer and to Enlightened Opinion* (translated by A. R. Price & V. Woollard). London: Karnac.

Miller, J. -A. (2006). Lacan, pour de vrai. *Le Monde des livres*, 20 January.

Miller, J. -A., & Etchegoyen, H. (1996). *Silence brisé: Entretien sur le mouvement psychanalytique*. Paris: Agalma/Seuil.

Miller, J. -A., & Milner, J. -C. (2004). *Voulez-vous être evalué?* Paris: Grasset.

Milner, J. -C. (1989). *Introduction à une science du langage*. Paris: Seuil.

Milner, J. -C. (2002). *Le périple structural: Figures et Paradigme*. Paris: Seuil.

Misès, R. (2005). À propos de l'expertise Inserm relative au *Trouble des conduites chez l'enfant et l'adolescent. La lettre de psychiatre française, 149*: 13–15. Available at: www.spp.asso.fr/Main/Actualites/.

Money-Kyrle, R. E. (2001). An inconclusive contribution to the theory of the death instinct. In: M. Klein, P. Heimann, & R. Money-Kyrle (Eds.), *New Directions in Psychoanalysis* (pp. 499–509). London: Tavistock, 1955 [reprinted Abingdon: Routledge, 2001].

Norcross, J. C. (Ed.) (2002). *Psychotherapy Relationships that Work*. New York: Oxford University Press.

Orrigi, G., & Sperber, D. (2004). A Pragmatic Perspective on the Evolution of Language and Languages (translated by M. Lieberman). Available at: www.interdisciplines.org/coevolution/papers/6.

Pelc, I. et al. (2005). *Psychothérapies: définitions, pratiques, conditions d'agrément, (avis n° 7855 du Conseil Supérieur d'Hygiène)*, June. Available on the website of the Service public fédéral (SPF) Santé publique, Sécurité de la Chaîne alimentaire et Environment.

Perron, R., Brusset, B., Baruch, C., Cupa, D., & Emmanuelli, M. (2004). Quelques remarques méthodologiques à propos du rapport Inserm "Psychothérapie: trois approches évaluées". *Bulletin de la Société Psychanalytique de Paris, 73*: 118–125. Available at: www.spp.asso.fr/Main/Actualites/Items/24.htm.

Pham, T. (2005). Outils d'évaluation chez l'adulte. HAS, *Prise en charge de la psychopathie*, pp. 31–34.

Pignarre, P. (2001). *Comment la dépression est devenue une épidemie*. Paris: La Découverte & Syros, Hachette Littératures.

Pinker, S. (2006). Block that metaphor! *New Republic*, 9 October. Available at: http://www.newrepublic.com/authors/steven-pinker.

Plantade, A. (2004). Lettre ouverte au Prof. Brechot, directeur de l'Inserm. Available at: forumdespsychiatres.org.

Pommier, G. (2004). *Comment les neurosciences démontrent la psychanalyse.* Paris: Flammarion.

Quine, W. V. (1953). Two dogmas of empiricism. In: *From a Logical Point of View* (pp. 20–46). Cambridge, MA: Harvard University Press, 1961.

Radtchenko, A. (2005). *Abstract Psychiatrie,* Issue 9, September.

Renik, O. (2003). Standards and standardization. *Journal of the American Psychoanalytical Association,* 51, supplement: 43–55; reprinted in *Fort-Da,* 2005, *11*: 60–72.

Rizzolatti, G., Fogassi, L, & Gallese, V. (2001). Neurophysiological mechanisms underlying the understanding and imitation of action. *Nature Reviews Neuroscience,* 2: 661–670.

Rodriguez Del Barrio, L., Corin, E., Poirel, M. -L. (2001). Le point de vue des utilisateurs sur l'emploi de la médication en psychiatrie: une voix ignorée. *Revue Québécoise de Psychologie,* 22 (2): 201–223 Available at: www.rrasmq.com/Publications.html.

Rodriguez Del Barrio, L., Bourgeois, L., Landry, Y., Guay, L., & Pinard, J -L. (2005). *Repenser la qualité des services en santé mentale dans la communauté.* Sainte-Foy (Quebec): Presses de l'Université du Québec.

Rose, S. (2005). Will science explain mental illness? *Prospect,* 115: 28.

Sackett, D. L., Straus, S. E., Richardson, W. S., Rosenberg, W., & Haynes, R. B. (1997). *Evidence-Based Medicine: How to Practice and Teach EBM.* Edinburgh: Churchill Livingstone.

Schmidt, E., & Cohen, J. (2013). *The New Digital Age: Reshaping the Future of People, Nations and Business.* London: Hodder & Stoughton.

Scott, P. (2000). The impact of research assessment exercise on the quality of British science and scholarship. *Anglistik,* 1: 129–143.

Shapiro, D. A., & Shapiro, D. (1982). Meta-analysis of comparative therapy outcome studies: a replication and refinement. *Psychological Bulletin,* 92 (3): 581–604.

Shapiro, D. A., & Shapiro, D. (1983). Comparative therapy outcome research: methodological implication of meta-analysis. *Journal of Consulting and Clinical Psychology,* 51 (1): 42–53.

Sheely, G. (1999). *Hillary's Choice.* New York: Random House.

Simon, H. A. (1969). *The Sciences of the Artificial.* Cambridge, MA: MIT.

Smith, M. L., & Glass, G. V. (1977). Meta-analysis of psychotherapy outcome studies. *American Psychologist,* 32: 752–760.

Solms, M. (1997). *The Neuropsychology of Dreams: A Clinico-Anatomical Study.* Mahwah, NJ: Erlbaum.

Solms, M. (2004). Freud returns. *Scientific American,* 290 (5): 82–88.

Sonenreich, C. (2004a). Psiquiatria sem evidências. *Newsletter do Projeto Análise,* 4 July. Available at: www.jorgeforbes.com.br.

Sonenreich, C. (2004b). Sobre a MBE. *Newsletter do Projeto Análise,* 2 April. Available at: www.jorgeforbes.com.br.

Spielberg, S. (2002). *Catch Me If You Can*. DreamWorks.

Srinivasa Murthy, R. (Ed.) (2001). Solving mental health problems. Chapter Three in *Mental Health: New Understanding, New Hope*. Geneva: World Health Organization. Available at: www.who.int/whr/2001.

Strathern, M. (2000). The tyranny of transparency. *British Educational Research Journal*, 26 (3): 309–321.

Strupp, H. H., & Hadley, S. W. (1979). Specific vs nonspecific factors in psychotherapy. *Archives of General Psychiatry*, 36: 1125–1136.

Swendsen, J. (2004). Lettre adressée aux enseignants en psychopathologie des universités françaises. 2 March, unpublished.

Szasz, T. (1957). On the theory of psychoanalytic treatment. *International Journal of Psycho-Analysis*, 38 (3/4): 166–182.

Thurin, J.-M. (2004a). Text posted at: www.techniques-psychotherapiques.org.

Thurin, J.-M. (2004b). A propos de l'expertise collective Inserm sur l'évaluation des psychothérapies. Text posted at: www.techniques-psychotherapiques.org, 26 February.

Thurin, J.-M. (2005a). Programme collaboratif de recherche sur le traitement de la dépression. Text posted at: www.techniques-psychotherapiques.org.

Thurin, J.-M. (2005b). Une évolution de la conception de la pratique basée sur la preuve à l'Association Américaine de Psychologie (APA). Available at: www.techniques-psychotherapiques.org.

Tsoukas, H. (1997). The tyranny of light: the temptations and paradoxes of the information society. *Futures*, 29: 827–843.

Turing, A. (1937). On computable numbers, with an application of the *Entscheidungsproblem*. *Proceedings of the Mathematical Society*, 2 (42): 230–65 [see also *errata* in 2 (43): 544–6].

Tyson, P. (2004). Review of *Affect Regulation, Mentalization and the Development of the Self* by Fonagy, P., Gergely, G., Jurist, E. L., & Target, M. *Journal of the American Psychoanalytic Association*, 52 (2): 631.

Valéry, P. (1951). Notes on the greatness and the decadence of Europe. In *Reflections on the World Today* (translated by F. Scarfe). London: Thames and Hudson.

Vasseur, C. (2004). La psychothérapie et la loi, ça marche ... sur la tête! Posted on the website of the Association française de psychiatrie (AFP).

Victorri, B. (2007). *Homo narrans*: the role of narration in the emergence of human language (English version). Available at: hal.inria.fr/docs/00/15/37/24/PDF/Narrative.pdf [original French version in *Langages*, 2002, 36 (146): 112–25].

Wampold, B. E. (2001). *The Great Psychotherapy Debate: Models, Methods and Findings*. London: Routledge.

Wampold, B. E., Mondin, G. W., Moody, M., Stich, F., Benson, K., & Ahn, H. (1997). A meta-analysis of outcome studies comparing bona fide psychotherapies: empirically, "all must have prizes". *Psychological Bulletin, 122* (3): 203–215.

Westen, D., Novotny, C. M., & Thompson-Brenner, H. (2004). The empirical status of empirically supported psychotherapies. Assumptions, findings, and reporting in controlled clinical trials. *Psychology Bulletin, 130* (4): 631–663.

Widlöcher, D. (1996). *Les nouvelles cartes de la psychanalyse.* Paris: Éditions Odile Jacob.

Widlöcher, D. (2004). N'en faisons pas un saint. Interview with Marie Huet. *L'Express*, Issue 2773, 23 August.

Wilson, M. (2003). The analyst's desire and the problem of narcissistic resistances. *Journal of the American Psychoanalytic Association, 51* (1): 71–99.

World Health Organization (1994). *The ICD-10 Classification of Mental and Behavioural Disorders.* Geneva: WHO.

Zagury, D. (2005). L'expertise pénale des psychopathes. HAS, *Prise en charge de la psychopathie*, pp. 128–129.

INDEX